CONTENTS

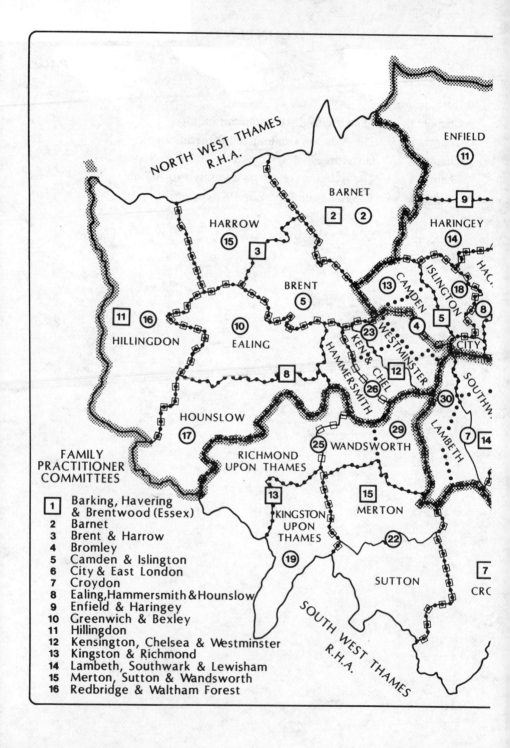

NORTH WEST THAMES R.H.A.

ENFIELD
⑪ 11

BARNET
2 ②

HARROW
⑮ 3

HARINGEY
⑭

BRENT
⑤

⑬ CAMDEN ISLINGTON ⑱
13 5 8 ⑧

11 ⑯
HILLINGDON

EALING
⑩

23 WESTMINSTER
KEN & CHEL ④ 5
HAMMERSMITH 12
26 CITY

SOUTHW.

8

HOUNSLOW
⑰

30
29

LAMBETH
7 14

25 WANDSWORTH

RICHMOND UPON THAMES

FAMILY PRACTITIONER COMMITTEES

13 KINGSTON UPON THAMES

15 MERTON

⑲ 22

7 CRO

SUTTON

1	Barking, Havering & Brentwood (Essex)
2	Barnet
3	Brent & Harrow
4	Bromley
5	Camden & Islington
6	City & East London
7	Croydon
8	Ealing, Hammersmith & Hounslow
9	Enfield & Haringey
10	Greenwich & Bexley
11	Hillingdon
12	Kensington, Chelsea & Westminster
13	Kingston & Richmond
14	Lambeth, Southwark & Lewisham
15	Merton, Sutton & Wandsworth
16	Redbridge & Waltham Forest

SOUTH WEST THAMES R.H.A.

PRIMARY HEALTH CARE IN THE INNER CITIES AFTER ACHESON

GERALD RHODES

USHA PRASHAR, KEN YOUNG

Foreword by Brian Abel-Smith

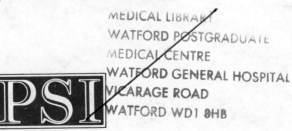

PSI Research Report No. 653, September 1986

Sales Representation: Frances Pinter (Publishers Ltd).
Orders to: Marston Book Services
P.O. Box 87
Oxford OX4 1LB

PSI Reports are available through all good bookshops, or in case of difficulty from PSI, 100 Park Village East, London NW1 3SR.

ISBN 0 85374 363 0

Printed by Blackmore Press,
Longmead, Shaftesbury, Dorset

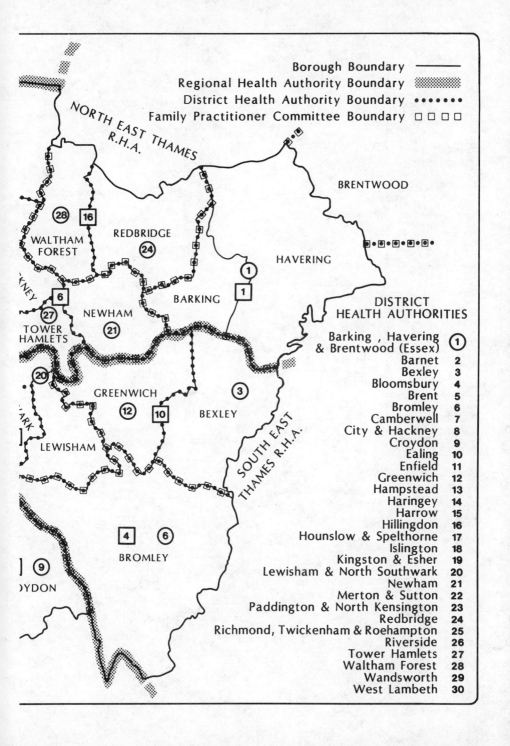

Borough Boundary ——
Regional Health Authority Boundary ░░░░
District Health Authority Boundary ••••••
Family Practitioner Committee Boundary ☐ ☐ ☐ ☐

NORTH EAST THAMES
R.H.A.

BRENTWOOD

㉘ 🔟16

REDBRIDGE

WALTHAM
FOREST

㉔

HAVERING

🔟6

NEWHAM

BARKING

🔟1
🔟1

㉗

㉑

TOWER
HAMLETS

㉒0

GREENWICH

🔟10

BEXLEY

③

LEWISHAM

⑫

SOUTH EAST
THAMES R.H.A.

🔟4 ⑥

BROMLEY

🔟9

DYDON

DISTRICT
HEALTH AUTHORITIES

Barking , Havering
& Brentwood (Essex) ①
Barnet 2
Bexley 3
Bloomsbury 4
Brent 5
Bromley 6
Camberwell 7
City & Hackney 8
Croydon 9
Ealing 10
Enfield 11
Greenwich 12
Hampstead 13
Haringey 14
Harrow 15
Hillingdon 16
Hounslow & Spelthorne 17
Islington 18
Kingston & Esher 19
Lewisham & North Southwark 20
Newham 21
Merton & Sutton 22
Paddington & North Kensington 23
Redbridge 24
Richmond, Twickenham & Roehampton 25
Riverside 26
Tower Hamlets 27
Waltham Forest 28
Wandsworth 29
West Lambeth 30

FOREWORD

This is the story of a government promise which did not materialise. London primary health care problems 'had been left unresolved for too long' Ministers told the House of Commons in January 1980. The government was going 'to put something into rapid and effective action'. Such were the brave words of new and inexperienced Ministers in the early days of office—impatient to pull the levers of power if only they were told which levers to pull. The Acheson Committee's task was to identify the levers. Only sixteen months later, 115 levers were specified. It took the government two and a half years to make a token response, and a further two and a half years to publish the long promised Green Paper, diluted by this time to an agenda for discussion 'long on items for discussion but not on firm proposals', as *The Times* correspondent put it. Action had been neither rapid nor effective.

The issue of the quality of primary health care is of critical importance for health care and recognised to be so internationally. As the World Health Organisation has pointed out, primary health care is the key to achieving Health for All by the Year 2000. It is important in two different ways. First, it is the base for personal curative, preventive, promotional and rehabilitative services. Second, a strong system of primary health care can prevent the over-use of hospital services—very much a London problem—and thus go a long way towards containing health care costs in the long run. This later point could be expected to appeal to a government pledged to hold down public expenditure not just in the short run but in the long run.

Why then did government fail to make more than a token response to Acheson? The King's Fund London Committee, which had with its limited funds supported a series of innovative schemes to indicate what might be done on a wider scale, felt that this question needed to be answered in depth. Hence it commissioned this study from the Policy Studies Institute. It was felt that understanding the real obstacles to change would stimulate thought about how they could be overcome. It was also felt that the issues raised by the Acheson report were too important to be allowed to be forgotten.

As the PSI study shows, governing is difficult. (Reigning, if tedious at times, is somewhat easier.) The conflicting objectives of governments have somehow to be reconciled. The interests of different groups in society (often the powerful few and the powerless many) have to be balanced. What might help a government achieve its long-run aims has to be weighed against the short-term political cost of resolute action.

Change, if it is to be relatively painless, generally costs money. The last major change in primary health care—the doctors' charter of 1966—needed not a little money to oil its wheels. It also needed considerable political courage to force it through without a major disruption of services. Money has not been available to DHSS Ministers in the 1980s to sweeten any pills they may have wished general practitioners to swallow. It was, of course, open to Ministers to force general practitioners to retire at 70 without compensation, to make the saving of paying full basic practice allowances for 1,500 patients rather than 1,000 in order to help finance an extra capitation fee for registering new patients, and give less remuneration to general practitioners working outside the inner cities so as to give more to practitioners working within them. But to act in this way might well have brought the general practitioner service into the same sorry state as the education service. And the sums of money needed for the government to buy its way out of trouble were not small, as what was done for London would have had to be done for other inner cities.

The political cost of a disrupted general practitioner service had to be weighed against the political gain of a better primary health care service. Dissatisfaction with primary health care was not, however, the cause of inner city riots. It is, however, true that many Londoners—particularly new Londoners—were experiencing difficulties in finding a general practitioner who would enlist them and in contacting their practitioner if they had succeeded in finding one. It is true also that many practitioners operated from shoddy premises, but patients were free to look for something better if they did not like what they had 'chosen'. The dissatisfied customers were not politically mobilised, however, or readily mobilisable: they were disproportionately the poorer section of society, the ethnic minorities, the unsettled and mobile without a community base.

The main arguments for improving primary health care, however, were technocratic arguments rather than responses to consumer complaint. To say this is not to belittle them but to explain the lack of a strong local constituency of political support. Continuity of care, integration of curative and preventive services, the creation of primary health care teams, even the take-up of preventive services are not issues on which local communities will man the barricades. In these circumstances it is not surprising that small numbers of conservative but articulate doctors could frustrate long-term improvements in health favoured not only by virtually all political parties but by the Royal College of General Practitioners.

This is not to say that the Acheson Report had no effect. But, as the PSI researchers show, improvements were slow, local, uneven and unco-ordinated. While the big issues were not tackled, many small reforms were on a piecemeal basis. Some family practitioner committee administrators, with the support of stronger lay committee members, dared to probe and attempted to act on sensitive issues such as the use of deputising services, the quality of premises and catchment areas. Attempts were made to improve local co-ordination between community health services, family practitioner services and social services departments despite the chaotic boundary mess of London with its new districts, older boroughs, ancient regions and the redundant areas which FPCs now serve alone—the residue of integration failure despite the pronounced policy objectives of successive governments and the upheavals of successive reorganisations.

This study explains why bold promises were broken. More is needed to govern than good intentions. Hopefully its analysis will help some government some day to heal the sores which have for far too long been festering within our National Health Service. It would be sad if Britain, once the leader, became overtaken by country after country in Europe as they rush to put into practice the policy of Health for All based on effective, accessible and acceptable primary health care.

Brian Abel-Smith
June 1986

INTRODUCTION

The publication of the report of the Study Group on Primary Health Care in Inner London (the Acheson Report) in May 1981 was an important event for many people concerned with the problems which it discussed. This was certainly true of the King's Fund which, four months after the report was published, held a conference to discuss the issues raised and, in particular, practical ways in which its recommendations might be implemented[1].

At that time there was some expectation that the government might make an early response to the report. In the event, it was another two years before it announced a series of measures for which special funding of £9m was to be provided, spread over three years. These measures, announced in October 1983, were not, however, confined to London but were to benefit other inner cities as well. Many of them derived from recommendations in the Acheson report, but some did not. On the other hand, a number of important recommendations which required action by the government for their implementation were not referred to at all in this package of measures.

The government had also, at the time when the report was published, commended it particularly to regional and district health authorities and to family practitioner committees for action, since many of the detailed recommendations were directed at these bodies. Health authorities and family practitioner committees thus had a dual role to play in responding both to the 'Acheson money' provided as a result of the October 1983 announcement and to the detailed recommendations.

Concern was, however, expressed by the King's Fund and particularly by members of its London Project Executive Committee at the inadequacy of the response to the Acheson report, and especially at the fact that after two and a half years the government had failed to deal with some of the more important issues raised. The Fund therefore approached the Policy Studies Institute with a view to initiating a research project which would not only examine the nature of the response and why it took the form it did, but would also consider what lessons, general or particular, could be learned from such a study which could have a bearing on the future development of primary health care policy.

After discussion between the two bodies it was agreed that to make sense of the response to the Acheson report it would be necessary, first, to examine

1

the origin of the inquiry, and, secondly, to analyse the nature of the study group's approach as reflected in its report. Examination of response to the report also seemed to require a dual approach. It was clearly important to try to elucidate why the government had taken so long to respond to the report and why its eventual response took the form it did. It was equally important to try to see what impact the report had had on the regional and district health authorities and family practitioner committees who were having to cope from day to day with the problems of providing primary health care in inner London.

This then in outline is what we have attempted to do in the following pages. We do not claim to have provided a definitive answer to the question 'what difference has the Acheson report made?' Rather, we have tried to draw out of the analysis the factors which seem to be of most significance for the future development of primary health care in inner London, and, indeed, for reasons which are fully discussed later, in the inner cities generally.

The research could not have been carried out without the full co-operation of many people who consented to be interviewed and provided essential information. They included members of the study group, officials of the DHSS and many people working for health authorities and family practitioner committees. We are greatly indebted to them and others for the time and effort which they gave to helping us. Needless to say, they bear no responsibility for the views expressed.

We should also, on behalf of PSI, like to express our thanks to the King's Fund London Project Executive Committee for commissioning this study, and to Jane Hughes and Pat Gordon among its staff for making our task easier.

Ken Young had overall responsibility for the project at PSI and the detailed research was carried out by Usha Prashar and Gerald Rhodes.

Reference
1 *Primary Health Care in Inner London*, Report of Conference at the King's Fund Centre, 22 September 1981, KF Report KFC 81/206.

2

CHAPTER 1   THE ORIGINS OF THE ACHESON INQUIRY

Introduction

Most committees of inquiry have an identifiable immediate origin and a more or less lengthy background history which may not always be easy to elucidate but which nevertheless may have considerable significance both for the way in which the committee approaches its task and for the subsequent reception of its report. The Acheson inquiry, although seemingly limited to a narrow investigation into primary health care in inner London, had an unusually complex background history, as well as a fairly obvious immediate origin. Both will be traced in this chapter.

In seeking answers to the question why the provision of primary health care services in inner London should be thought to raise such problems as to merit a special inquiry, one has to look at three inter-related aspects: developments in the NHS generally; developments affecting health care provision in the conurbations and especially inner city areas; and developments specifically affecting London.

As a preliminary to this analysis, it may be noted that, although the Acheson inquiry functioned and was generally treated as being a committee of inquiry, it was in form simply a study group of an ad hoc advisory body, the London Health Planning Consortium; and that although it was concerned only with inner London, its report has proved significant in relation to the problems of primary health care in inner cities generally. Both these aspects will be further discussed later.

Developments in the National Health Service

This is not intended to be a history of the National Health Service, but certain developments of the last 20 years, especially those affecting the primary care services, are important for an understanding of the work of the Acheson inquiry.

A useful starting point is the dissatisfaction within the medical profession in the 1960s which led the British Medical Association's General Medical Services Committee (GMSC) to put forward a plan for considerable changes in the way general practitioners were paid, and for improvements in their conditions of service. This new 'charter' did not propose any change in the fundamental

3

position of GPs as 'independent contractors' to the NHS, but it did set its sights on some improvements which have remained topical since, such as the need for more ancillary staff and for the modernisation and improvement of premises; and it argued that it was essential for the government to provide greater inducements in under-doctored and 'special' areas[1].

The government, after negotiation with the GMSC, accepted a large part of the charter proposals. Of particular relevance here is the fact that it was agreed to provide positive financial incentives to doctors working in areas which, largely on the basis of figures of average list size, were held to be short of doctors. In these designated areas a special allowance was to be payable to all general practitioners[2]. Another of the GMSC's proposals, that an independent body should be set up to finance the purchase and modernisation of doctors' premises, was also accepted[3].

The 1960s and early 1970s were also a time when much emphasis was given to the problems of organising primary health care, meaning essentially those services provided in the community mainly in contrast to the hospital services. Until the reorganisation of the National Health Service in 1974 responsibility for primary health care was split between health and local authorities. Nevertheless, the idea gained ground that the most effective way of organising primary health care was through a team which would include doctors and nurses and possibly other professions too. Both the Royal College of General Practitioners[4] and the BMA[5] endorsed this approach, and certainly in pre-reorganisation days the most common form of team working was through the attachment of local authority nursing staff to doctors' practices[6]. For many people team working was associated with group practice of GPs, and largely for other reasons there had since 1948 been a considerable move away from single-handed towards group practice. More controversial was the ideal arrangement, as seen by some, of teams working in health centres, that is, specially designed premises provided by local authorities or, after 1974, by health authorities.

The 1974 reorganisation brought the community health services which had formerly been the responsibility of local authorities under the newly created area health authorities (AHAs), but general practitioner services continued to be separately administered by family practitioner committees (FPCs). The need for closer working between the different parts of the NHS, which was one factor in the plans for reorganisation, was, however, only partly met by bringing the financing of the administration of FPCs within the responsibility of AHAs.

Planning and management issues were perhaps the most prominent of those which had led to reorganisation becoming a live question in the 1960s. But planning focussed attention on problems of resource allocation. These had become evident as a result of the introduction of the comprehensive Hospital Plan of 1962. The fundamental problem was that the system of allocation was not based on an assessment of the needs of different areas, taking into account any changes which were taking place, but was largely determined by the existing pattern of distribution, often going back many years. After an unsuccessful attempt to devise a formula which would help to allocate resources more equitably in 1970, the whole subject was referred to a Resource Allocation Working Party (RAWP) in 1975.

The RAWP was required to suggest a method of allocating resources to regions and areas which would ensure that they corresponded 'objectively, equitably and efficiently to relative need'. The working party was concerned only with resources going to health authorities. It could not, therefore, consider the resources provided through FPCs for the family practitioner services. These were based to a large extent on demand for the services in question. The working party did, however, suggest that there should be a review of financial interactions between health authority and FPC services[7].

The formula suggested by RAWP was adopted by the government. Its implications for London will be discussed later. Meanwhile, two other initiatives by the Labour government elected in 1974, although not directly connected with the decision to set up the Acheson inquiry, were of relevance to the problems of providing primary health care. A Royal Commission on the National Health Service was appointed in 1976 with wide-ranging terms of reference. Although it did not issue its report until shortly before the decision to set up the Acheson inquiry in 1979, it might have been expected to, and did, draw attention to many of the issues which were prominent in the Acheson discussions. The second initiative was much more closely concerned with the development of primary health care. The question of priorities within the health service was explicitly raised in a consultative document issued in 1976. This proposed considerable expansion of primary care services, and particularly of the health visitor and home nursing services, as a means, among other things, of relieving pressure on the hospital services, by far the most expensive part of the NHS[8]. This was part of a generally changed emphasis on providing care for particular groups such as the elderly and the mentally ill as far as possible in the community rather than in hospital.

One cannot, however, leave this sketch of health service developments which had a bearing on the setting up of the Acheson inquiry without drawing attention to the financial constraints which have restricted the NHS, as they have other aspects of public expenditure, since the mid 1970s. In particular, the system of cash limits on expenditure, first introduced by the Labour government in 1976 but much extended and strengthened by the Conservatives in 1981, not only compelled closer attention to value for money in health care but made more difficult the introduction of innovations which, as is usually the case, were likely to increase the cost of services. Increasingly, and inevitably, the development of the NHS has taken place against a background of often fierce arguments about whether the NHS is being unduly affected by these financial constraints or whether it is at least able to meet adequately basic demands made on it. These disputes have, however, been most evident in the period since the Acheson committee reported, and the consequences for the reception of that report are, therefore, discussed later in this study.

Cash limits have, however, only been applied to the expenditure of regional and district health authorities. Expenditure on the administration of FPCs is, therefore, restricted in this way[9] but not the substantial payments made to doctors, dentists etc. for the services they provide under contract to the FPCs. As might be expected, this contrast between health authority and FPC expenditure has attracted the attention of the Treasury, but again this belongs mainly to the post-Acheson period.

The broad conclusions which can be drawn from this background have been well summarised by Professor Alan Maynard. He points out that in the period of rapid expansion of expenditure on health care in the 1960s and early 1970s the emphasis was on inputs—more doctors, more nurses, more beds etc. This approach came increasingly under question as pressure on the use of resources grew. At the same time there was more detailed questioning of equity issues in RAWP as well as the attempt to define priorities[10]. What seems evident is that the result of these tendencies was to shift attention away from the hospital sector to some extent and more towards primary health care. Initiatives such as the Hospital Plan of 1962 seem to epitomise the expansionist era in which the cost of the family practitioner services formed a decreasing proportion of total NHS expenditure. The 1976 discussion document on priorities and other developments around that time, of which the appointment of the Acheson committee forms a part, are an indication of the need that was seen to pay more attention to primary health care. It was not so much a concerted change of direction but rather a result of a number of disparate factors tending to point in the same direction: changing views on patient care combining among other things with the realisation of the daunting costs of hospital care in a population with an increasing proportion of the elderly provide one example. This shift must not be exaggerated. Expenditure on the Family Practitioner Services represents only about 20-25 per cent of total NHS expenditure, and although this does not constitute the whole of expenditure on primary health care the hospital services are likely to continue to attract most attention, just as they attract the major part of professional prestige. What has happened is simply that there has been more realisation that the contribution of the primary health services must not be neglected. One consequence has been to draw greater attention to the problems of providing effective primary care, not least in the inner areas of London and other big cities.

Primary health care in the inner cities
Certain problems of providing primary health care in inner city areas had long been evident. Provision of adequate premises, progress in establishing group practices or setting up primary health care teams, ability to attract high quality general practitioners, recruiting and training (and retaining) sufficient district nurses and health visitors, these were all matters in which it seemed that inner cities often had greater difficulties than other areas. In many cases these problems had a long history. Before the NHS was established, the strength of the teaching hospitals and the policies they followed (for example, provision of free outpatient departments) tended to weaken general practice in inner city areas. Beyond that, there was the question of whether the characteristics of the population of these areas might impose a greater workload on those doctors who did practise there; for example, a higher incidence of certain diseases

might be expected in run-down areas inhabited largely by those with ill paid jobs or, increasingly, no jobs at all.

The medical profession was not slow to draw attention to the problems. An editorial in the *Journal of the Royal College of General Practitioners* in 1972, for example, declared that:

> organising good primary care in big cities is more difficult than arranging good specialist care[11].

Four years later it suggested 'the problems are getting worse . . . something has got to be done' [12].

In 1977 the Minister of State with responsibility for health matters (Mr Roland Moyle) acknowledged that the GMSC had for years been drawing attention to some of the difficulties which general practitioners faced in inner city areas[13].

An obstacle to rapid progress in dealing with these problems was the fact that frequently the remedies proposed involved greater expenditure on primary health care in the inner cities. This was true of the BMA's charter proposals of 1965 with their incentives for doctors to practise in under-doctored areas. Although something was done on these lines, it was not sufficient to make any real impact on what was increasingly felt to be a deteriorating situation.

Health care was, however, only one part of a general problem posed by declining areas in the centres of big cities, and it seemed as though any attempt to tackle primary health care problems might need to be linked with more general policies for the inner cities. That at least could be one reading of the situation when the Labour government brought out its White Paper of 1977 which put forward the concept of a partnership between central government and certain local authorities as a means of trying to improve social and environmental conditions in the areas worst affected.

So far as health care was concerned, there was an obvious difficulty in that a partnership between central and local government left relatively little scope for improvement of health services and particularly family practitioner services. Perhaps not surprisingly the White Paper was somewhat vague on the subject of health beyond saying that in partnership areas health authorities would be brought into the local machinery[14]. But, no doubt as a result of the interdepartmental discussions which preceded the publication of the White Paper, the DHSS was stimulated into giving a good deal more prominence to the issue of primary health care in the inner cities. In particular, a series of papers produced by the Department formed the basis of discussions with representatives of the GMSC and the RCGP in November 1977.

These papers, and parallel papers dealing with nursing, were in theory concerned with primary health care in the conurbations generally but the discussions in fact centred on the inner city areas of those conurbations. This does, however, draw attention to one of the most prominent underlying themes affecting the whole debate, and of particular importance for discussion of the Acheson report. The question was how widely inquiries should go. Did conurbations have problems of a distinctive kind from the rest of the country, or was it simply that it was the inner city areas which required special attention? And was inner London merely one example of the inner cities, or did it have particular problems calling for special examination? And if it did, could inner London be regarded simply as one entity, or did the problems vary to such an extent within inner London that different areas had different needs? These were not just academic questions but had very definite practical consequences especially when it came to deciding what, if any, additional resources needed to be applied to the improvement of primary health care[15].

The papers which formed the basis of the 1977 discussions drew attention to ways in which statistically the conurbations, and more particularly London, differed from the rest of the country: for example, the percentage of single-handed practitioners was generally greater, and in Greater London much greater, than in England and Wales as a whole; large lists were common, except in London; fewer health centres had been built than in the rest of the country; there were more elderly doctors than in the rest of the country. Other information related more specifically to the inner areas of the conurbations; for example, areas having lower than average ratios of health visitors and district nurses to population tended to be found there.

On the question of what was to be done about the problems of providing primary health care which lay behind such statistics, the DHSS in the working papers listed suggestions which had been made without comment beyond noting that some of them would require the allocation of resources on a scale which was unlikely to be feasible. The immediate outcome of the discussions seemed to be a rather indefinite promise of future action: 'further thought', for example, was to be given to ways of attracting and retaining nursing staff. For the rest, the views of the representatives of the medical profession were noted: for example, that there was a need to attract well trained young practitioners to the inner cities, and that it was both 'practicable and desirable' to provide health care there through primary health care teams. And among the means by which these ends were to be attained, the idea of special financial incentives to practise in inner city areas was prominent[16].

No doubt other ideas came out of these discussions. It was later claimed, for example, that the idea of a GP 'facilitator', that is, a GP specially appointed for an area to visit local GPs to give help and advice on such questions as the improvement of premises, was suggested by Sir Henry Yellowlees, the Chief Medical Officer at the DHSS, at these discussions[17]. And two further inquiries carried out jointly by the DHSS and professional representatives owed something at least indirectly to these 1977 discussions. The first of these was indeed referred to by the Secretary of State (Mr David Ennals) in a somewhat inadequate reply to the Opposition spokesman (Mr Patrick Jenkin) about what he was doing to remedy the deficiencies of general practice in cities. Among other things, he said, a joint working party to include also representatives of the Society of Family Practitioner Committees was being set up to consider the problems of under-doctored areas[18].

The term 'under-doctored areas' derived from the criteria adopted by the Medical Practices Committee for classifying areas for the purpose of deciding whether to accept or refuse applications to practise, and in particular to the use of average list size. An area was classified as 'designated' and needing more doctors on the basis that average list sizes were large, that is, above a specified figure. Designation was, however, increasingly felt to deal with only one part of the problem of areas requiring more doctors; and in any case the number of designated areas was declining. From over 300 in 1970 it had dropped to seven in 1983. The terms of reference of the working party therefore went beyond designation and required it to consider 'what characteristics determine whether there are sufficient general medical practitioners in an area'. Moreover, it was to look at the factors, financial and non-financial, which affected under-doctored areas, and to suggest criteria for identifying them and measures to try to get enough doctors into them.

Again, it is significant that, although the terms of reference of the working party were quite general, Mr Ennals specifically included the establishment of the working party in a list of what was being done in connection with the inner cities. Designated areas were, however, not confined to inner city areas, and there were other reasons for the appointment of the working party. The whole system of classifying areas, linked, from 1966 onwards, with the payment of incentives, received criticism on grounds both of effectiveness and equity. Indeed the working party, in its report published just at the time when the Acheson study group was being set up, firmly concluded that it was inequitable to pay the additional practice allowance to all doctors working in an area with high average list size. Beyond this, the system did not in its view recognise that an area might need more doctors even though its figures of average list size did not reach the level adopted as a criterion by the MPC; social and environmental factors, it pointed out, might mean that those living in some areas had greater than average needs and provided greater workloads for general practitioners. It recognised that in thus broadening the approach it was touching on the difficult subject of the quality of service provided, drawing a contrast between an area with a large proportion of elderly single-handed doctors in poor premises etc. with one with the same number of doctors but with a balanced age distribution, good premises and supporting staff[19].

In spite of this forthright analysis, the working party was unable to make any very positive proposals for effective action. It pondered over the question whether social or demographic indicators might be used in conjunction with list size to determine the need for general medical services, but 'with regret' it concluded that the practical difficulties were too great[20]. Nor had it been able to work out an alternative to the designated area allowance, perhaps based on a standing allowance together with increased capitation rates for doctors in under-doctored areas, although it hoped that something on these lines might be possible in the future[21]. Its main proposal was that the arrangements for paying initial practice allowance should be modified and be much more dependent on demand based on local consultation. It might seem from this analysis that the working party hardly merited much attention. The issues raised, however, the GMSC's reaction to the report, the Acheson study group's handling of the questions, and not least the continuing debate about them, all contribute to the need to see this as an important issue, particularly in relation to inner London.

The second inquiry which may be seen as having indirectly sprung from the 1977 discussions was of a very different nature. It will be recalled that in the 1960s and 1970s the concept of the primary health care team as the most effective means of providing such care had gained increasing acceptance, and had been advocated by the medical profession in the 1977 discussions for the inner cities in spite of the obvious practical difficulties of organising such teams there. Towards the end of 1978, however, the Secretary of State's Standing Medical and Nursing and Midwifery Committees set up a joint working group to consider the problems of establishing and running primary health care teams. This working party, under the chairmanship of Dr Wilfrid Harding, was again of a general nature, but its report makes clear that a major reason for the inquiry was that in some areas, particularly inner cities, it was thought that, for financial and other practical reasons, enthusiasm for the concept of the primary health care team was waning and schemes of attachment of nursing staff, for example, were being abandoned. It is not surprising, therefore, that, although most of the report was taken up with a discussion of the general issues involved, a number of specific recommendations were made in relation to the problems of team work in declining urban areas. Since, however, the working group was still in operation at the time of the establishment of the Acheson study group, and indeed its report was published on the same day as that of the study group, further reference to its work will be made later.

But did anything more positive and immediate come out of the discussions between the DHSS and the profession? Writing to the *British Medical Journal* in 1981 after his retirement, one of the senior medical officers of the DHSS who had been involved in the discussions admitted that finance was the principal reason why so little progress had been made[22]. The point was taken up more bluntly in the medical profession. At the annual conference of Local Medical Committees in 1978 a resolution was passed that the GMSC should press the DHSS to introduce direct funding of primary health care in certain deprived areas[23]. Commenting on this one medical journal suggested that it was frustration and anger within the profession over the lack of government action which had 'exploded' at the conference, because:

> despite a succession of promises from Ministers, little progress has been made in achieving a formula for attracting young family doctors into the nation's older cities or for providing them with adequate practice premises[24].

Seven months later a writer in another journal was still bemoaning the fact that fifteen months after the 1977 discussions: 'nothing much seems to have happened'[25].

Again, the 1979 LMC conference passed a resolution regretting that the chief medical officer had still: 'failed to produce concrete proposals for an improvement in the quality of primary health care in the conurbations'[26].

Dire warnings over the years from the GMSC that services might break down in inner city areas if nothing was done made little impression if, as a prominent member of the GMSC claimed, the DHSS insisted that any improvement must come from existing budgets[27]. And while it was unlikely that any 'new money' would be forthcoming for this purpose in 1978, the possibility diminished further in May 1979 with the election of a Conservative government pledged to exercise tight control over, and reduce, public expenditure. Moreover, it was not clear whether inner city problems would have a high priority for the new government. Following the election, a comprehensive review of inner city policy was instituted which put the future of the urban aid programme in doubt.

Nevertheless, the Royal Commission, reporting shortly after the election and therefore reflecting conclusions arrived at before it, added its voice to those urging that additional financial resources should be provided to improve primary health care services in declining urban areas, declaring roundly that:

> in some declining urban areas and in parts of London in particular the NHS is failing dismally to provide an adequate primary care service to its patients . . . improving the quality of care in inner city areas is the most urgent problem which NHS services in the community must tackle[28].

In spite of this, there was considerable doubt by the time that the Acheson study group came to be appointed at the end of 1979 whether decisive and effective action to deal with the problems of providing primary care in inner urban areas could be expected. The importance of the subject ensured, however, that pressure was maintained by articles in the medical press and in other ways from the profession, with practical suggestions being put forward which led to a good deal of controversy[29]. Moreover, one issue continued to exercise the GMSC. Its chairman might, understandably, say of the working party on under-doctored areas that it was:

> a difficult working party to serve on[30]

but the issues raised there, and particularly the recognition of the fact that an area might lack sufficient doctors even though the average list size was not particularly high, were clearly ones which the GMSC wanted to pursue.

About the time that the Acheson study group was being set up, the GMSC appointed a working group mainly to consider reaction by LMCs to the working party's report. It concluded that the working party was wrong to argue that it was not possible to identify under-doctored areas (or rather under-privileged areas, a more appropriate term favoured by the working group) by objective criteria. The group then examined this question further as well as the related question of providing financial and other incentives to attract doctors into such areas. A preliminary report was produced in 1980 recommending that special allowances and payments should be made to doctors working in under-privileged areas, provided that satisfactory criteria could be established for identifying such areas. Further research was proposed for this purpose[31]. All this was of course going on, like the work of the Harding working group on primary care teams, at the time when the Acheson study group was carrying out its task.

One other development in the late 1970s which, although not directed specifically at the inner cities had clear implications for the provision of medical care in them, needs also to be mentioned here. In 1977 a body with the unusual title of a 'research working group' was set up by the DHSS to examine a question which had long troubled many people concerned with the provision of health care: the difference in health standards experienced by people in different circumstances. The most striking example, and one which had been commented on long before the NHS was established, was the difference in mortality rates of different social classes. The task of the working group, under the chairmanship of the Department's chief scientist Sir Douglas Black, was primarily to analyse available information and indicate the causes of differences in the health experience of different social classes or the need for further research. But such an immense task could hardly be undertaken without drawing implications for policy. It is not surprising that the group took three years to produce its report which was published shortly after the Acheson study group had begun its work. Among other things it advocated a very large shift of resources within the NHS towards community care as a means of attempting to break the links between social class and illhealth[32].

Health services in London
The preceding section has suggested that during the 1970s there was much concern that it was becoming increasingly difficult to provide adequate primary health care services in many inner city areas. This situation had been brought about chiefly by social and economic changes which altered the composition of the population living in inner city areas, and which at the same time made it difficult both to provide suitable premises and to attract and retain adequate medical and nursing staff for what were often problem areas for health care as for other services. To the extent that inner London shared these characteristics it might be thought that practical proposals for dealing with the problems of providing primary health care in inner cities could be applied to London as much as to Liverpool or Birmingham. Yet not only was a specific inquiry instituted in 1979 into inner London's primary health care problems but this followed shortly after the Royal Commission's recommendation that there should be an urgent inquiry by an independent body into a whole range of problems affecting the provision of health services in London, that is, not confined to primary health care nor to inner London[33].

The need for such a wide-ranging inquiry was summarily rejected by the government[34], but the Royal Commission's discussion of this issue does suggest that it is important to make clear what were the special problems of London and how these affected more specifically primary health care in inner London. It should then be possible to assess how far distinctive features of the London scene, rather than the features it had in common with other cities, contributed to the decision to set up the Acheson study group.

The Royal Commission suggested four major areas requiring detailed examination in London:

the administration of post-graduate teaching hospitals;
whether London needs four regional health authorities;
whether special adjustments to the RAWP proposals are needed to take
account of the concentration of teaching hospitals in London;
what additional measures can be devised to deal with the special difficulties of providing primary care services and joint planning[35].

The first three of these items draw attention to distinctive features of the
administration of health services in London which can in fact be traced back to
certain historical developments which accompanied the growth of London,
particularly in the nineteenth century. The wealth and size of London were a
major reason for the establishment from the eighteenth century onwards of a
comparatively large number of hospitals which in time became noted as centres
of teaching as well as treatment, attracting through their prestige many leading
members of the medical profession to work there.

These hospitals were concentrated in the area which from 1889 onwards
was known as the County of London but more particularly in the central areas
of the county. In the early part of the nineteenth century this was London and
the hospitals were situated in places which at least bore some relation to the
distribution of the population they served. By the end of the nineteenth century
this was ceasing to be true as London spread further into the surrounding counties[36]. In the period since 1945 the continuing decline of population from the
LCC area has raised even more sharply the question of whether the area is
overprovided with acute hospital beds largely in the teaching hospitals.

There have been other consequences of the existence of the teaching hospitals in central London. When the NHS was created in 1948 London was
carved into four segments for the purpose of the regional administration of
hospitals. A major reason was the fact that it was not possible, as in the prov-
inces, to create RHB areas on the basis of one or two teaching hospitals at the
centre. A single RHB for London would have been unbalanced in having a
large part of the country's teaching hospitals in one region. Nevertheless, the
existence of four RHBs (or, since 1974, four RHAs), each consisting of a segment of inner London plus a segment of outer London and a part of the Home
Counties, poses problems for any attempt to examine and plan for developments affecting the whole of London.

Equally, it is often argued that the way in which the teaching hospitals
developed in London weakened the development of the general practitioner
services[37]. The argument is that the quality of the hospitals and their accessibility to the local population led to reliance on them for services which elsewhere
were much more likely to be provided by GPs. This is suggested as one of the
factors which contributed to there being by the 1970s more elderly single-
handed GPs with small lists in inner London that in the country generally, and,
more significantly, than in other inner city areas.

Thus in a sense two linked questions, the position of the teaching hospitals
and the organisation of the NHS in London generally, marked the distinctive-
ness of London from the rest of the country. One obvious consequence was

that, to the extent that problems arose which affected London as a whole, there was no administrative mechanism within the NHS which could formulate policies to deal with them. Some ad hoc mechanism had to be devised in which, inevitably, much depended on initiatives from the centre, since the DHSS was the only authority which could effectively bring together the various interests involved.

Attempts at co-ordinating a London approach were indeed a feature of the 1950s and 1960s[38] but several factors made the situation more urgent in the 1970s. Administratively, the fact that the teaching hospitals were brought under the RHAs in 1974 almost inevitably led to closer attention being paid to the question of whether there was an imbalance between the provision of acute hospital beds in inner London as compared with outer London and indeed the outer areas of the four Thames RHAs. At the same time, the implementation of the RAWP proposals in 1976 put particular pressure on the Thames regions, since a major feature of the RAWP formula was that it provided for more of the total of resources available to be allocated to regions like Trent and North West than had been the case under the previous system, and less to other regions, particularly the four Thames regions. When this formula was applied, as was increasingly the case from the late 1970s onward, with tight control of total expenditure on the NHS, the effect was to make even more acute the dilemma for each of the Thames regions of how to allocate the resources made available to them among the various competing claims.

It may be that as a result, as has been claimed:

> in London (where the problem is obviously most acute) it has required the health authorities to make decisions about the balance between teaching hospitals and other services that should probably be taken nationally[39].

Nevertheless, even without national decisions on such questions there were clearly problems which affected London as a whole and which could not be resolved simply by each RHA taking its own decisions without reference to the other three. Much therefore turned on the nature of any initiatives taken by the DHSS to try to put these problems into a broader context.

The White Paper on reorganisation of the NHS had committed the government to taking some action on this question[40], but it was during the time when Dr David Owen was Minister of State at the DHSS (1974-76) that there was particular pressure for action to be taken over the problems of health care in London. In 1975 a London Co-ordinating Committee was established under the chairmanship of the Permanent Secretary of the Department, Sir Patrick Nairne. Its main object was to explore the degree of common ground which existed among the various authorities concerned with health problems.

The committee was not a success. After the first year or so it hardly met. Various explanations have been suggested for this lack of success among those closely involved with the committee. It was a large and somewhat diffuse body with representatives from such diverse authorities as the RHAs and the London Boroughs' Association. It tended to be too politicised, with members more concerned with defending their particular interests than with trying to find compromise solutions to problems. It lacked an agreed basis from which to start examining those problems.

The failure of this initiative put pressure on the DHSS to find some more effective way of getting some kind of agreement on what needed to be done in London. Within the DHSS, liaison with NHS (and local) authorities in the regions was the responsibility of the two Regional and Planning Divisions until 1976 when it became the responsibility of a single Regional Liaison Division. London co-ordination was one responsibility of the Regional and Planning Division but it was not closely associated with the London liaison work. For example, in 1975 one Branch was concerned with liaison with the NE Thames, NW Thames and East Anglia Regions, another with liaison with the SE Thames, SW Thames, Wessex and South Western Regions, and a third with London co-ordination, relations with London University and various general responsibilities. The 1976 reorganisation of responsibilities within the DHSS also brought about a much closer concentration on London issues, with a single Branch now having responsibility both for liaison with all four Thames Regions and for co-ordination of NHS planning for London.

The Under Secretary in charge of the Regional Liaison Division from 1976 to 1978 and subsequently, until his retirement in 1980, of one of the two RL Divisions into which it was split in 1979 was Mr J.C.C. Smith. Much of the credit for further initiatives on London problems belongs to him, although Mr Roland Moyle, who became Minister of State in 1976 and was himself a London MP, backed the continuation of the Owen policy. J.C.C. Smith, variously described by colleagues who had worked with him as having an entrepreneurial flair and a gift for getting hold of the right staff for his division at the right time, seems to have drawn the lesson from the failure of the Co-ordinating Committee that it was better to proceed in two stages: first, to get agreement as far as possible in a smaller, tighter and less politically dominated body on what needed to be done; secondly, to seek the endorsement of these proposals by a high-powered advisory group.

This was the origin of the London Health Planning Consortium (LHPC) established in 1978, and of the London Advisory Group (LAG) set up two years later. Given the nature of the London health, and particularly hospital, scene, the strategy favoured by Smith required a good deal of preliminary persuasive work to get its acceptance by the various divergent and powerful interests involved. In effect, the membership of the Consortium consisted of four elements: the four RHAs; the University Grants Committee; the University of London; and of course the DHSS itself. Smith was chairman, and the RHA members were a carefully mixed group of regional administrators, medical officers, nursing officers and treasurers. The letter with which Smith announced the appointment of the Consortium said that other bodies would be brought into its discussions when matters affecting them were involved.

The terms of reference of LHPC were:

to identify planning issues relating to health services and clinical teaching in London as a whole; to decide how, by whom and with what priority

15

they should be studied; to evaluate planning options and make recommendations to other bodies as appropriate; and to recommend means of co-ordinating planning by health and academic authorities in London.

The introductory letter of the chairman, although couched in diplomatic language, suggested a determined and clear idea on his part of the direction in which he hoped the Consortium would go. After making it clear that the LHPC was neither a decision making nor an executive body, the letter stressed that anything put forward whether as analyses, proposals or advice, would need to be the subject of formal consultation and decision by Ministers and the statutory authorities. Nevertheless:

it is already clear that high priority needs to be given to the problems of matching teaching with service needs and to the scale and pattern of provision in some medical specialties.

The letter also mentioned the proposals to set up 'a small Advisory Group of eminent persons' to advise the Secretary of State, since some issues might:

call for decisions of major significance for London, and indeed the country as a whole[41].

On the face of it, this seems a fairly complex piece of machinery for resolving London's problems, and one which could lead to delays in reaching decisions. On the other hand, there were many links between LHPC and the London Advisory Group set up later; for example, whereas LHPC had senior officers from the four Thames regions as members, LAG had all four regional chairmen. Above all, there was the link provided by the DHSS, not least in the secretariat of the two bodies. One can only conclude that the DHSS was driven to this mechanism largely because of the failure of the London Co-ordinating Committee, hoping that agreement in LHPC and endorsement by LAG would generate a certain momentum for action. It was an optimistic approach, given the history of attempts to deal with London's health problems.

Over a year after the LHPC was set up, and while it was actively engaged in preparing its first major consultation paper, the Royal Commission on the National Health Service published its recommendation for an independent inquiry into London health problems. It is hardly surprising that, having embarked on a quite different course for dealing with those problems, the government rejected the recommendation. Nevertheless, the Commission's proposal does raise the question of why investigation of London's health problems took the form it did. One strand in the answer has already been referred to in the need to find something more effective than the Co-ordinating Committee, but in wider terms the answer must derive from the peculiar structure of the NHS.

It has been noted that, although health authorities are appointed bodies, and not, like local authorities, elected, there are often great difficulties in securing that national policies and priorities are carried into effect in the NHS[42]. Hence it is natural that the DHSS should seek to make progress by somehow carrying along with it those bodies which in the end are largely going to determine by their actions whether national policies are actually carried into practice. In a similar way much investigation into health service problems derives from the work of committees of inquiry appointed by the various standing committees which advise the Secretary of State on medical matters, rather than from ad hoc committees of investigation, such as indeed the Royal Commission of 1976-79 was[43]. In this sense LHPC and LAG, although unusual in form, can be said to owe their origin to the distinctive nature of the administrative structure of the National Health Service.

There were perhaps other factors too. The particular nature of the London teaching hospital problem meant that both the University Grants Committee and London University and not simply the health authorities would be closely involved in any decisions which would need to be taken[44]. Again, to single out London for examination by an ad hoc committee of inquiry might have been politically difficult, given the strongly held view of the BMA in particular that other inner city areas such as Liverpool presented equally severe problems for the provision of health care. A purely advisory body, like the LHPC, limited to the consideration of issues which arose out of developments peculiar to London, was not so liable to come up against objections of this kind.

At all events, the Consortium soon got down to the major and intractable problem of the future pattern of acute hospital services in London. Its first publication did not suggest how that problem should be resolved. Rather, in accordance with J.C.C. Smith's step-by-step approach, it was a rather glossy publication, described as a 'profile'. It was not a plan, but:

at best it is intended to provide an indication of the direction in which planning may need to proceed[45].

This kind of 'softening up' approach was further emphasised in the conclusions which, after boldly stating that the distribution of acute hospital services in the Thames regions was 'decidedly out of balance' with the distribution of population, drew the facts set out in the document to the attention of:those who need to address themselves to the task of providing well balanced health care and related services in London and the South East of England[46].

After thus preparing the way, the LHPC went on to formulate more positive proposals in a discussion document which did not shirk controversy; it suggested, for example, that the future of Westminster Medical School was in doubt[47]. What is important, however, is that the whole argument in the document was based on an analysis of the need for acute hospital beds, the methodology of which had been devised by the Consortium itself. This pragmatic approach, looking at needs and then relating them to the existing pattern of hospital services without regard to administrative boundaries, was a characteristic strength of the LHPC's work. It made it less easy to dispute the extent of reduction in acute hospital beds which was needed, although there could, of course, still be plenty of argument about the implications for particular hospitals and especially for individual teaching hospitals. In this latter context, the controversial Flowers report largely reinforced the LHPC's work.

There is no doubt that this major issue on which the Consortium concentrated its efforts became increasingly the focus of public attention as closures of beds, wards or even complete hospitals began to be carried out in the late 1970s and early 1980s. It was not, however, the only concern of the LHPC. It set up subgroups to examine the distribution of beds for a number of specialties, and produced factual 'profiles' of a number of specific patient groups, for example, the mentally ill. The question of finding ways to improve the provision of primary health care in inner London also arose at an early stage. From what was said earlier it might be thought that this issue would in any case have been raised in its own right, but undoubtedly what gave urgency to it was the fact that it was indissolubly linked with the major question of the provision of acute hospital beds. For if it was true that the growth and prestige of the teaching hospitals in the inner areas of London had inhibited the development of primary care services so that hospitals had assumed a role there which elsewhere was the function of the primary care services, then a major reduction in the provision of hospital beds such as was clearly intended by the Consortium would, unless remedial steps were taken, expose further inadequacies in the existing primary health care services.

In fact, the Consortium, as in its examination of the hospital sector, attempted to analyse what was happening in primary health care, taking in not only questions like the extent to which cases were dealt with by hospital accident and emergency departments which should have been dealt with by general practitioners, but also broader issues such as the reasons why London medical graduates were not anxious to go into general practice in inner London. In thus trying to define the problem more precisely the Consortium almost inevitably took into account some factors which were mainly or entirely of significance in London and some which London shared to a greater or lesser extent with other inner city areas. The difficulty for the Consortium was to find a way of dealing effectively with the primary health care problems which it had defined. It did not itself have particular expertise in primary health care because its immediate concern had been with the hospital bed situation, and its membership had been chosen with that in mind. Nor was it in a position to make good the gaps in the available data which a recent inquiry by the Royal College of General Practitioners had revealed[48].

The solution adopted was to commission an inquiry by a specially constituted study group, whose membership was drawn from the various interests concerned with primary health care in London but with an independent chairman. It was to make recommendations to the Consortium which would itself then advise its constituent bodies, including the DHSS; and even then no action was likely until the LAG had added its advice. Formally, therefore, the study group added yet another layer to the decision-making process. The reality was rather different. There was no overlap of membership between LHPC and the study group, and in practical terms the latter was a body appointed by and reporting to the Secretary of State, the LHPC having only a nominal role. As with LAG, the important link was with the DHSS, especially through the secretariats of the various bodies.

One last point needs to be made here. The study group was not formally appointed until January 1980 but the essential strategy for its appointment had been agreed before the general election of May 1979. The need to get the endorsement of the new Conservative Ministers led to some delay, but the strongest argument in favour of an inquiry, and one which would report reasonably quickly, was that a reduction in acute hospital beds would have to be balanced by improved primary care. How this was to be done seemed an urgent question.

Summing up

A simple answer can be given to the question 'what was the origin of the Acheson study group?', or a much more complicated one. The simple answer derives from the logic of the imbalance of hospital beds in the Thames regions. To have accepted the case for a reduction in beds in inner London without examining the consequences for primary health care would have been at the least bad planning. From that point of view it is hardly surprising that the LHPC, a body, as its name indicates, which had as its primary aim the consideration of planning issues, should from the beginning have seen the future of the primary health care services as one of its tasks. The link between primary and secondary services was clearly strong and perceived as such by the LHPC. Yet it was the urgent need to deal with the question of the imbalance of acute hospital beds, with its particular consequences in inner London for the teaching hospitals, which was the immediate and precipitating factor for the inquiry into primary health care.

In other words, the focus here is on the local nature of the issues, and the fact that, without the immediate problems over acute hospital beds, it is unlikely that there would have been an inquiry into primary health care in inner London. The immediate cause of the setting up of the Acheson study group is, therefore, clear enough. It will, however, be one of the themes of this study that neither the work of the study group nor the reception of its report is intelligible unless one takes into account the wider context within which it operated. This is a much more complex area, but two main strands can be identified. The first is the increasing concern with primary care generally, particularly after the shift in government policy foreshadowed in 1976 in *Priorities for Health and Personal Social Services*. If primary care was to help relieve pressures on the hospital service then it was essential to ensure that it could do this effectively, in inner London as elsewhere. Hence, the various examinations of aspects of primary care such as the Harding working group on the primary health care team.

The other main strand was the recognition of the special problems of providing primary health care in certain areas. As earlier discussion has made clear, inner city areas were a major element in this but they were never the whole of it. The concepts of under-doctored and under-privileged areas, as well as more general concern with the social and environmental problems of inner city areas, ensured that there was much analysis of the difficulties of providing primary health care services in the inner cities and of what needed to be done to overcome those difficulties.

There was thus a certain ambiguity in the origins of the Acheson study group. There were clearly immediate London problems, and these were reflected in the terms of reference of the Acheson inquiry. But what those terms of reference did not recognise was that it might not be meaningful to deal with London's problems in isolation, and that their examination might raise the kind of wider issues about providing primary health care in inner cities which have been referred to earlier. The history of London's health service provision might differ in some important ways from that of Birmingham or Manchester, but there could be no doubt that London shared with other cities some of the problems of providing adequate primary health care, just as it shared with those cities many of the characteristics of urban decline. How far London was unique, and how far the group's work was applicable only to London, then become relevant issues in the wider context. It will be argued in later parts of this study that these questions are of fundamental importance in understanding both what Acheson did and what action followed its report.

References
1   See 'A Charter for the Family Doctor Services', *British Medical Journal*, Supplement, 13 March 1965.
2   This was in addition to the initial practice allowance given, for the first three years only, to doctors setting up in a designated area; this had operated since 1948. On this, see John R. Butler, *Family Doctors and Public Policy*, Routledge and Kegan Paul, 1973, Ch.1.
3   The General Practice Finance Corporation was established under the National Health Service Act 1966.
4   *Present State and Future Needs of General Practice*, RCGP, 1970.
5   *Report of Working Party on Primary Medical Care*, BMA, 1970.
6   This had been recommended by a sub-committee of the Minister's Standing Medical Advisory Committee in the 1960s. *The Field of Work of the Family Doctor*, HMSO, 1963.
7   *Sharing Resources for Health in England*, HMSO, 1976, para.6.21.
8   *Priorities for Health and Personal Social Services in England*, HMSO, 1976, p.2 and para.3.12.
9   From 1 April 1985 FPCs have become completely independent of DHAs and directly accountable to the Secretary of State, but their administrative costs are still subject to cash limits.
10   *Change: The Challenge for the Future*, RCGP, 1984, pp.13-14.
11   'Primary Care in Big Cities', *Jl. RCGP*, 22, 1972, pp.653-4.
12   'General Practice in Big Cities', *Jl. RCGP*, 26, October 1976, p.171.
13   *British Medical Journal*, 1 October 1977, p.908. The BMA were anxious to have this on record in view of the Minister's earlier criticism of poor surgery premises etc. in London. *British Medical Journal*, 4 June 1977, pp.1487-8.
14   *Policy for the Inner Cities*, Cmnd 6845, HMSO, 1977, Annex, paras.29-32.
15   Of particular importance was, and is, the attitude of the medical profession; the BMA, for example, through the GMSC, has consistently taken the view that it would be wrong to single out London for special treatment.
16   *On the State of the Public Health for the year 1977*, HMSO, 1978, pp.62-4.
17   Dr Arnold Elliott, in *Health Trends*, November 1984, p.74.
18   HC Deb. 14 November 1977, vol. 939, WA 55/6.
19   *Report of Working Party on Under doctored Areas*, DHSS, 1979, para.11. Earlier criticism of the effectiveness of the designated area allowance had led DHSS to commission a research project on the subject in 1968. See Butler, *op.cit.* who points out that the GMSC had a long-standing aim of directing extra resources to areas where there were high workloads rather than high average list sizes, (p.16.)
20   *Report of Working Party*, *op.cit.*, para.12.
21   *Ibid.*, para.19.
22   Dr Thomas E.A. Carr, *British Medical Journal*, 31 January 1981, p.403.
23   *British Medical Journal*, 22 July 1978, p.306.
24   *Pulse*, 8 July 1978, p.1.
25   Michael Lowe, 'DHSS wait on urban rot', *General Practitioner*, 2 February 1979, p.30.

26   *British Medical Journal*, 14 July 1979, p.158.

27   Dr Arnold Elliott in *Pulse*, 8 July 1978.

28   *Report of Royal Commission on the National Health Service*, Cmnd 7615, HMSO, July 1979, paras. 7.58, 7.62, 7.63.

29   See, for example, Michael Downham, 'Medical Care in the Inner Cities', *British Medical Journal*, 19 August 1978, pp.545-8; Brian Jarman, 'Medical Problems in Inner London', *JL RCGP*, October 1978, pp.598-602. The Conservative Medical Society issued a discussion paper in 1979 suggesting that DHSS might need to allocate specific funds for promoting primary health care teams in inner cities, *Primary Health Care in the Inner Cities, a blueprint for action*. The GMSC also, following further dissatisfaction within the profession over general practitioners' pay, produced a report which among other things stressed the need for financial incentives to attract GPs to 'areas of environmental and social deprivation', *Report of the New Charter Working Group*, BMA, February 1979, paras 12.2, 12.8.

30   *British Medical Journal*, 24 November 1979, pp.1380-3.

31   GMSC Report 1980, paras.120-4: 1981, paras.107-9. *British Medical Journal*, 27 September 1980, pp.883-5.

32   *Inequalities in Health*, DHSS 1980, para.8.24.

33   Cmnd 7615, para.17.18.

34   HC Deb. 23 January 1980, vol. 977, col.466.

35   Cmnd 7615, para.17.18.

36   Even in the early years of this century it was being remarked that there was a lack of balance between population and provision of hospitals in London. (See Geoffrey Rivett, 'The work of the London Health Planning Consortium', in King's Fund Project Paper, *London's Health Services in the 80s*, No.25, Pt 3, April 1980, p.45.)

37   cf. David Morrell, 'Inner London general practice: is there a solution?', *British Medical Journal*, 10 January 1981, p.162.

38   For example, four joint consultative committees were established by the metropolitan regions in 1965, and in 1967 a joint working party under the chairmanship of Dame Albertine Winner, a former Principal Medical Officer in the Ministry of Health, was concerned with London-wide co-ordination.

39   John R. Butler and Michael S.B. Vale, *Health and Health Services*, Routledge and Kegan Paul, 1984, p.84.

40   *National Health Service Reorganisation: England*, Cmnd 5055, HMSO, 1972, para.185.

41   *London Health Planning Consortium*, DHSS letter to London Regional and Area Administrators and Secretaries of Boards of Governors, 4 May 1978. The London Co-ordinating Committee was still nominally in existence at this stage, as a further complication in the machinery.

42   cf. Howard Elcock and Stuart Haywood, *The Buck Stops Where?*, Institute for Health Studies, University of Hull, 1980. Butler and Vaile, *op.cit.*, pp.86-7.

43   See Gerald Rhodes, *Committees of Inquiry*, RIPA/Allen and Unwin, 1975, pp.167-76.

44   London University set up its own inquiry in 1979 into the problems of medical schools, under the chairmanship of Lord Flowers: its report was published in 1980 as *London Medical Education A New Framework*.

45   *Acute Hospital Services in London*, HMSO, 1979, p.2.

46   *Ibid.*, p.32.

47   *Towards a Balance: a framework for acute hospital services in London reconciling service with teaching needs*. A discussion document issued by the London Health Planning Consortium, February 1980, paras. 41, 42, 56.

48   *A Survey of Primary Care in London*, RCGP Occasional Paper 16, 1981, attempted to bring together the available information.

CHAPTER 2 THE ACHESON COMMITTEE IN OPERATION

Introduction

The Acheson Study Group on Primary Health Care in Inner London[1] held its first meeting in January 1980 and published its report in May 1981. This chapter considers the way in which the committee approached its task and the nature of the report it produced. The object is not to discuss its findings in detail but rather to draw out the significant features of the committee's operation which may have a bearing on the way in which the report was received.

Some preliminary points need to be made. It was in the first place a comparatively large committee. This was mainly because of the need to make sure that the numerous interests involved in primary health care in London were given the opportunity to put their points of view. This did not mean that it was a purely representative committee. Members were chosen as individuals and some at least only agreed to serve on that basis, but at the same time, as commonly happens with committees, care was obviously taken to ensure that there was a wide involvement of those concerned with the provision of primary health care in London. If doctors were the most prominent group (9 of the 14 members excluding the chairman), they came from a variety of backgrounds, including general practice, community medicine, medical schools and LMC administration. There were in addition nurses, an FPC administrator and local authority officials. With such a diversity of points of view the choice of chairman was both difficult and crucial. Clearly someone of standing was required who was not identified with particular London interests or partisan solutions to the problems of primary health care there. The choice of Professor Donald Acheson, who then held the chair of Clinical Epidemiology at Southampton University, promised well. With a wide range of experience and interests but particularly in the community medicine field and NHS administration (through membership of a RHB and AHA), and as a leading figure in the world of academic medicine[2], he seemed an ideal choice for this difficult task.

The second general point about the committee concerns the expectations of those appointing it. The terms of reference were broad. It was to:

define the problems of organising and delivering primary health care in inner London in relation to medical and nursing services, taking into account existing and current studies; to identify the measures required to overcome these problems and to recommend, in order of priority, the actions which might be taken by the various bodies concerned; to identify which areas require further study, considering the way in which the studies might best be undertaken, and to make recommendations to the Consortium; and to consider specific matters remitted to it by the Consortium[3].

It is particularly interesting that the committee was asked specifically to take into account existing and current studies and also to list 'in order of priority' the actions to be taken by the various bodies to put into effect the recommended measures. To these need to be added the gloss put on the terms of reference by J.C.C. Smith in his introductory letter to Professor Acheson. Pointing out that much had already been written about the problems of providing primary health care services and of what might be done about them, Smith added 'regrettably little has happened'. What was needed, therefore, was particularly 'measures which could achieve change within a short timescale—say, five years'. On this basis Ministers—Dr Gerard Vaughan, the Minister of State for Health was specifically mentioned—were backing the inquiry and awaiting its report 'with considerable interest'. Finally the hope was expressed that the committee might be able to report by the end of 1980[4].

On the face of it, this suggests that what was aimed at was a quick inquiry drawing largely on work already done and making practical suggestions which could be put into effect straightaway. Certainly, this was the theme of ministerial pronouncements in the first months following the setting up of the Acheson inquiry. In January 1980 the Secretary of State, in rejecting the Royal Commission's call for a general inquiry into London health care problems as 'a recipe for delay', said that London's problems:

> have been left unresolved for too long. In the interests of Londoners and indeed of the rest of the country, the uncertainty must be ended and that is what we aim to do[5].

The Minister of State was more specific in the same debate:

> we have had a series of inquiries on London. What we need is some action.

After existing inquiries were completed, including Acheson, the government would:

> through a powerful London committee, put something into rapid and effective action[6].

Further elaboration of this theme was provided by the Minister of State in June 1980 in arguing against an inquiry into the possibility of creating a single RHA for Greater London. The Acheson inquiry had been instituted because of the lack of information on the primary sector, but once it had reported it would be the LAG's task to:

> pull together the various reports that are available[7].

These pronouncements have to be seen against the more general political background. The strategy for handling the planning and co-ordination of London health problems through the LHPC and LAG had, as has been seen, been devised under the Labour government. When that government was defeated at the May 1979 election it was likely that the incoming Conservative government would view it in a different light, especially given its commitment to reduce public expenditure. Although the Conservative election manifesto specifically excluded the NHS from spending cuts and emphasised the need for better use of existing resources, it was clear that proposals for increasing expenditure would receive very close scrutiny.

The decision to set up an inquiry into primary health care in inner London had been taken before the election. The incoming Conservative administration had no great enthusiasm for such an inquiry but probably found it easier to let it go ahead in view of its close link with the plans to reduce the acute hospital beds sector in London, provided that it did not raise too many awkward questions particularly in relation to the public expenditure commitment. Hence, the emphasis on a limited inquiry, and practical short-term measures drawing on existing work, made sense in that it made no commitment, and particularly no long-term commitment, but showed that the government viewed with some concern primary health care problems in inner London.

There were, of course, certain hazards in this approach. If a serious effort was to be made to deal with London's primary health care problems and to make an impact on them in the short term, it was hardly likely that there would not be some resource implications. Certainly, existing studies, such as those of the Royal Commission[8], almost all advocated additional financial resources. There was thus an implied commitment to providing additional resources for primary health care in the very fact of setting up the Acheson committee, but this did not raise serious difficulties at that stage when neither the scale of such resources nor the extent to which they could be provided from savings elsewhere could be predicted. Certainly, members of the committee at the beginning of their work did not have the impression that resource constraints were a serious obstacle.

The Acheson committee: general approach
Much, therefore, turned on the nature of the committee's inquiries and the scope of its recommendations. A key factor is the extent to which work already done or in process of being done provided an adequate basis for analysis of the problems and provision of solutions to them. Some of that work has been referred to earlier, including the Royal Commission and the working party on under-doctored areas. The Harding working group was also at work but its findings were not published until the Acheson committee had also completed its work. To these should be added a survey carried out by the International Hospital Federation in 1975 as part of a larger examination of primary health care problems in big cities; this raised questions about the financing and organisation of primary health care in London[9]. The RCGP inquiry was also

significant not least because of the links between it and the Acheson committee[10].

There were also a number of more localised studies such as the ambitious survey carried out by the Kensington, Chelsea and Westminster (South) CHC of attitudes to family practitioner services[11]. RHAs had examined the existing provision of primary care services and, to varying degrees, made plans for its development. One of the more extensive plans of this kind had been drawn up by the North East Thames RHA. And within the NE Thames area the Hackney/Islington partnership was one of the few such authorities to have made a close study of primary health care in its area. There was thus a good deal of information available about the situation in primary health care in London when the Acheson inquiry began its work in January 1980, and also no lack of suggestions for dealing with the problems revealed. The committee might therefore have chosen to review the literature, identify further information needed and elaborate possible solutions in discussion as necessary with those most closely concerned. Some such approach was implied in the ministerial and departmental views expressed at the time, with their emphasis on the need for speed and action. Yet even here there was ambiguity, again best expressed in the words of J.C.C. Smith's letter to Professor Acheson:

> The Consortium feels . . . that work is urgently needed both to draw out the suggestions from existing studies which are of greatest value and to recommend new lines of development and action . . .

> We have deliberately given the Study Group wide terms of reference so that you may be free to consider all aspects of the problems. Nonetheless, we regard it of the utmost importance to find solutions to which early effect can be given.

It seems as though two voices were speaking. The voice of those who conceived the study group as a wide-ranging inquiry, even though confined to London, and who saw the necessity of devoting additional resources to primary health care in the inner city was overlaid by the voice of those taking a narrower view after the 1979 election with its emphasis on short-term measures and more limited resource implications. The ambiguity was not resolved at the time of the committee's appointment, and was indeed probably a necessary feature of getting it established at all in the changed political circumstances brought about by the 1979 election.

Certain consequences were important for subsequent events. The committee undertook a wide-ranging inquiry and produced a report with over 100 recommendations for action, many of them requiring additional resources to be devoted to primary health care in inner London. Moreover, the request to concentrate on short-term measures was treated in a distinctly ambiguous fashion by the committee:

> we have not interpreted this to imply that we should be looking for short term solutions at the expense of long term need; our aim has been to make recommendations which would positively facilitate change rather than

(but not to the exclusion of) encouraging developments which might over a long period lead to change[12].

In thus aligning itself with the wider rather than the narrower approach the committee was doubtless influenced by a number of factors: the fact that a report based on a mass of evidence might make more impact and that unanimity among members of the committee might be helped by such an approach are perhaps two of the more important. It has to be remembered that, apart from the chairman, all the members of the committee were already deeply involved in the problems which they were being asked to resolve and tended to look at those problems from the point of view of their own experience of them. Professor Acheson was deeply committed to achieving a unanimous report, and weighty evidence could be seen as providing the basis of such unanimity or at least as exerting an educative effect on the members of the committee by involving them in a wider view of the problems and possible measures to combat them.

At all events, the scale of the committee's operation was very large. Not only did it invite evidence from all the health authorities and community health councils in the area[13], the local authorities, family practitioner committees and local medical committees and from professional and voluntary bodies and medical schools. It also wrote individually to all the GPs in London inviting their views. Nearly 200 individuals altogether, mainly doctors and nurses, provided their views in addition to the 175 responses from organisations. The scale of the committee's inquiry involved the DHSS in more administrative support than it had expected. Nevertheless, the Department appears to have accepted, initially at least, the need for an inquiry on this scale. Only later perhaps did misgivings arise as the implications, and particularly the financial implications, of the committee's approach began to emerge.

The pressure under which the committee and its staff worked can be judged from the fact that the report on primary health care in inner London was published only 16 months after the committee's first meeting[14]. This was, of course, longer than the optimistic 'before the end of 1980' target set more in hope than expectation by the Department but it represents a considerable achievement, given the decision to undertake a full-scale inquiry.

Many of the more important issues were the subject of much debate and argument in the committee before finally—with one exception—agreement was reached. Undoubtedly, the process of reaching agreement was helped by the fact that the need to work together in a committee exposed misunderstandings and ignorance of other points of view. This is a common enough feature of committees of inquiry but was particularly acute in a body like the Acheson committee. The clashes of personalities and ideas were reinforced by the quite different viewpoints from which individual members saw primary health care problems. A GP member whom others regarded as a diehard conservative in his views might see part of his task as being to educate his fellow members in what could realistically and practically be done. This is the kind of thing which goes on in most committees. But added to that were the vital elements in the primary care scene in inner London on which individual members brought quite specific experiences to bear. Did GPs appreciate as much as they should the role and problems of community nurses? Were single-handed GPs working in relatively comfortable areas aware of the difficulties of running a group practice in the more deprived areas? Before agreement could be reached a process of accommodation and mutual education on issues of this kind had to take place. If the committee itself took in evidence as widely as possible this might help to encourage the process to a greater extent than merely drawing on the inevitably selective material which happened already to have been produced.

Once having embarked on this course the main problem for the committee was how to keep its head above water. A vast amount of information and views poured in during the early months of 1980, ranging from half-page letters from some individual GPs to extensive memoranda from some of the main authorities and professional bodies. The aim here will be to try to see what the committee regarded as significant and how this influenced the shape of the report.

One clue to the committee's thinking lies in the choice of those questioned in oral evidence. They fall into three groups:

i) the main professional and similar bodies, such as the BMA, the Royal Colleges of General Practice, Nursing and Midwives and the Health Visitors' Association; to these may be added the Regional Medical Officers of the DHSS and, in view of the comparatively large number of doctors from abroad, the Overseas Doctors Association:

ii) the NE Thames RHA health care study group, the Hackney/Islington inner city partnership and the City and Hackney CHC;

iii) the Medical Directors Association and the Medical Practices Committee.

The first group is predictable and it would have been surprising if the committee, having decided to operate as a full-scale committee of inquiry, had not sought to examine further the views of these bodies beyond what they had provided in written evidence. The second group is less expected and indicates that the committee was impressed by what was happening and proposed in the north east corner of inner London. The third group seems at first sight rather surprising. The Medical Directors Association is a body representing many of those who provide deputising services for general practitioners, the MPC the statutory body with responsibility for influencing the distribution of GPs throughout the country.

Before attempting to see how the committee made use of the evidence presented to it some general points about its approach may be made. The report of the committee is long and closely argued, and covers a great variety of topics from the need for a retirement policy for GPs to the desirability of hospitals making their staff social and recreational facilities available to community nurses. There are, however, as one might expect, certain key points both in the analysis and in the recommendations which give the main clue to the committee's thinking. At the same time it must be said that in presentational terms the report makes no concessions to the reader. It is a solid document which requires a concentrated effort if the threads in the argument are to be fully appreciated. That, in itself, might not be very important but for the fact that the committee's terms of reference required it to indicate an order of priorities for action to be taken on its recommendations, and that has not been done explicitly but rather has to be inferred by the careful reader, picking his way through the 115 recommendations in all.

If one then asks how radical or conventional the committee was in its approach, the answer must be that it did not seek to alter fundamentally the system of providing primary health care in inner London, but that within the constraints which it accepted in its general approach it certainly felt free to make some controversial proposals, many of which, it must be added, did not fit easily with the expressed desire of the DHSS for more or less immediately practicable proposals. The most obvious point at which the question of a radically different approach arises is in the context of the status of general practitioners. Some would argue that the problems of providing primary health care in inner cities are unlikely to be resolved as long as GPs remain as independent contractors to the NHS, and the alternative most often canvassed is that of a salaried service. Neither this nor another suggestion sometimes made that hospitals should assume the main responsibility for primary care in inner cities received any discussion in the Acheson report, although it did recognise that in certain circumstances some kind of temporary or experimental arrangement on these lines might be desirable[15].

Nor did a salaried service or a hospital-based system of primary care figure prominently in the evidence to the committee, which was no doubt one reason why they were not discussed in the report. A more potent reason was that, given the composition of the committee, agreement on these issues would have been impossible, quite apart from the fact that, even if they had been put in the report, they would have aroused such opposition from the established interests that they would have had no chance of being put into effect. As one member of the committee put it, there was an unwritten agenda which did not include a salaried service because everyone realised that politically it was a non-starter.

The scope of the inquiry

Within these constraints the approach of the committee naturally fell into two parts: analysis of the problems; and suggestions for dealing with those problems. As to the first, little new could be expected; according to one member of the committee, the problems had been known for 50 years. Nevertheless, although many articles and reports had listed those problems, much turned on exactly how they were presented and especially on the relative importance given to different aspects. The committee right at the beginning of its report made a crucial distinction between problems springing from the needs of the population and those deriving from the difficulties of providing adequate services to meet those needs. And it is significant that the first chapter of the report deals with social and environmental conditions in inner London.

This emphasis undoubtedly owes a good deal to the fact that one member of the committee, Dr Brian Jarman, was deeply concerned with the problems of deprivation in London and their relation to the provision of primary health care[16], although of course some of the evidence drew attention to this wider context within which the provision of primary care services had to be considered[17].

Nevertheless, inevitably the greater part of the report is concerned with the way in which primary care services were being provided in inner London and with suggestions for improving that provision. One other general point needs to be made about the 115 recommendations listed at the end of the committee's report. Given the broad-ranging nature of its inquiry, it is hardly surprising that these were not wholly or even mainly short-term in scope. In fact they ranged from fairly simply changes which could be put into effect without much delay (information on answering machines to be displayed in doctors' surgeries, a simpler explanation of the General Practice Finance Corporation's cost rent scheme to be prepared, etc.) to measures which might require a certain amount of negotiation but could theoretically be brought in quite quickly (independent assessors to advise on appointments to single-handed vacancies, surgeries to comply with minimum standards to qualify for rent and rate reimbursement, etc.) and to others which not only raised major policy issues but whose effects would need to be measured over a longer period (retirement policy for general practitioners, the DHSS to institute a system of central funding for community nurse training, etc).

Much evidence to the committee was concerned with immediate and experienced practical difficulties. From the patient's point of view, for example, problems of registration with doctors or of accessibility and availability once a place had been secured on a doctor's list were a prominent feature; for doctors, problems of parking and, for nurses, transport problems generally were often mentioned. The committee did make practical recommendations on points like these but at the same time it also looked for what might be the underlying difficulties of which these could be symptoms. Registration and accessibility problems, for example, were seen as partly due to the characteristics of the population of certain parts of inner London, and partly to the structure of general practice there.

Nor was the committee content simply to add the evidence received to existing studies. In a number of cases it carried out, or asked others to carry out, surveys which it was hoped would establish the nature of some of the problems more precisely. The difficulties of registration, for example, were examined through information specially obtained from the deputising services and from certain Accident and Emergency Departments[18]. Furthermore, the findings from these necessarily small-scale studies led the DHSS, at the committee's suggestion, to commission a more extensive survey from the Office of Population and Census Surveys whose findings were published at a much later date[19].

From what has been said earlier, it is clear that the relative importance of the committee's many recommendations is not immediately obvious from reading its report. The analysis of the problems is lucid and the measures suggested to deal with them are on the whole presented in a reasoned and persuasive manner. But within each area of discussion recommendations are set down without any indication of priorities. Two reasons may be suggested for the committee's failure to identify priorities, as required by its terms of reference. There was, first, the difficulty of getting agreement within the committee. All could agree that the many measures proposed would contribute to the aim of improving primary health care, but members might differ considerably in the extent to which they attached importance to particular measures. This was clearly the main reason which influenced the committee in not attempting to put forward priorities. Secondly, it might be argued that in any case the interdependence of at any rate the major recommendations was of more importance than trying to establish priorities among them.

Even so, much can be inferred from the report itself about priorities. The largest single section relates to the general practitioner services, itself an indication that this was seen as a priority area by the committee. Within the section on general practitioner services, however, there are several strands. One priority which may be deduced is that of attracting more young GPs to work in inner London. The thought behind this was not that young doctors were necessarily better but that they were more likely to be committed to the idea of group practice and the concept of the primary health care team which, in common with much orthodox medical thinking, the committee accepted as being desirable goals so far as the organisation of primary health care was concerned. The other side of this equation, however, was that the committee identified the high proportion of elderly single-handed doctors in inner London as a major obstacle to the achievement of the aim of attracting more young doctors. Again, this was not because they were necessarily inferior doctors but simply that by temperament and training they were less likely to be attracted to the idea of group practice and teamwork.

The view that inner London needed to attract more young doctors was not novel and it figured prominently in some of the evidence to which the committee attached importance, such as that from the NE Thames RHA. However, the implications of trying to achieve this aim, and especially of linking it with the need to reduce the number of single-handed elderly practitioners, involved the committee in making recommendations over a wide area. Here, for example, the position of the MPC was seen as a vital one and hence the committee thought it necessary to take oral evidence from it. It was true that the MPC could not positively do much about attracting young doctors to inner London, but through the rules it used for classifying areas and through the guidance it gave to FPCs it might have a considerable influence on the structure of general practice. One point here was that length of general experience as a doctor carried considerable weight when appointments to single-handed vacancies were being considered, and this was in accordance with the views of the profession as expressed by the GMSC. Some departure from this attitude would, therefore, be needed if more opportunities were to be open to young doctors. The importance of the whole issue to the committee accounts for the considerable discussion in the report of the position of the MPC and also for the decision, surprising at first sight, to take oral as well as written evidence from the MPC.

To a large extent the committee was here concerned with the negative side of the problem of attracting young doctors, the obstacles which might prevent such doctors, however keen they were to practise in inner London, from having the chance to do so, whether because there were not enough vacancies or because when there was a vacancy existing rules and conventions made it difficult to secure appointment. The committee was haunted by the existing structure of general practice, and particularly the age structure. Following the more detailed pattern of the Jarman report[20], published figures showed that there were three times as many elderly doctors in inner London as in the country as a whole, with some parts of inner London having even higher proportions. Given the committee's assumption that the ideal to be aimed at was the primary health care team, even the sceptics on the committee became convinced that something needed to be done about the situation when the evidence showed that so many of these doctors were working in complete isolation both from other doctors and from other primary care services[21]. If sufficient elderly doctors could be induced or encouraged to cease practising then the prospects for attracting younger doctors would be much improved. But how was this to be done? A critical passage in the report argues the need for a rapid change in the situation and comes down in favour of a retirement policy for general practitioners rather than the removal of administrative restraints as a means of creating a comparatively large number of vacancies within a short time[22].

As the committee recognised, retirement policy was a national, and highly controversial, issue. It is not surprising that, as one member put it, the committee had 'interminable discussions' on it; nor that it produced more general arguments to show that a retirement policy was desirable on grounds other than the creation of vacancies for young doctors in inner London. Nor, perhaps, is it surprising that this issue broke the otherwise remarkable consensus within the committee on what needed to be done; Dr John Oldroyd dissented both from the concept of a retirement policy and from the views of the rest of the committee on the likely consequences of introducing such a policy[23].

What is clear, however, is that the committee gave high priority to attracting doctors, and particularly young doctors, to inner London. It was drawn into retirement policy and other controversial national issues, such as advocating a London weighting for GPs, as a means to that end. Yet the overriding need was the commitment to group practice and the concept of a primary health care team. This is evident in the discussion of premises, another topic to which the committee devoted a lot of attention. Of course, provision and maintenance of premises to a good standard could be seen as a desirable object in itself, but it was essential to make progress on this front if there was to be any chance of making the goal of team working a reality. This too was linked to the idea of attracting young doctors, since difficulties in obtaining suitable premises could act as a deterrent.

The other main aspect of the provision of general medical services discussed by the committee is not so directly related to the central theme of encouraging the primary health care team. A good deal of evidence, particularly from CHCs[24], related to difficulties of patients in getting access to GP facilities and to problems of availability of GPs. This involved the committee in considering, first, why some people failed to register with a doctor, and, secondly, what kind of arrangements doctors made to enable patients to make contact particularly outside surgery hours, involving the use both of answering machines and of deputising services. Once again, the committee did not confine itself to specifically London answers but raised national issues when, for example, it suggested that accessibility could be improved if GPs received a special fee on registration of a new patient[25].

The controversial issue of the use of deputising services again illustrates not only involvement in national issues but also the importance of the evidence in influencing the committee. It seems originally to have taken a fairly critical line in relation to the use of deputising services and it was for this reason that it took the apparently surprising step of taking oral evidence from the Medical Directors Association. In fact, the evidence impressed the committee, and although it did suggest some tightening of the administrative arrangements for controlling the use of these services, the report generally accepted the need for them[26].

In contrast to the lengthy analysis and urgency of its recommendations in relation to the general medical services, the remainder of the committee's report seems to lack the same depth. The community nursing services receive, after the general medical services, the most sustained treatment, but it is hard not to feel that the committee did not attach quite the same importance to the problems which they raised. For this there are a number of reasons. The committee was of course heavily weighted in favour of the medical profession, and much of the evidence concerned the problems of the general medical services; furthermore, such evidence as there was on the nursing services failed to make a strong impact on the committee. Moreover, there were few studies in existence specifically of the nursing services. Certainly, the impression is that the nursing members of the committee had a hard task in attempting to convince the other members that community nursing was also an urgent area. Beyond this, however, was the undoubted fact that if the problems of the general medical services could not be resolved it was unlikely that whatever was done on the nursing services would make a significant impact on the standards of primary health care in inner London.

Nevertheless, there were, as the committee recognised, difficult problems in the provision of adequate community nursing services in inner London. In analysing these problems it leaned heavily on work already carried out in the NE and NW Thames RHAs[27]. Its recommendations for the most part can be described as sensible, practical remedies to overcome the obstacles identified: provide nurses with cars and clerical assistance, make available to them hospital social and recreational facilities, etc. In going beyond this, in two ways it raised much wider issues, first, by recommending that the DHSS should institute a system of central funding for nurse training to overcome the disadvantages of inner London districts in having to sponsor a large number of students; secondly, in raising the whole question of the adequacy of the existing system to relate establishment levels to the workloads which nurses had to perform.

Of the other aspects of primary health care considered by the committee, little need be said. Perhaps the most important of these aspects concerned primary health care education where the committee came out quite strongly in favour of strengthening academic departments of general practice and postgraduate training. There were also a number of recommendations designed to improve organisation and management in primary care, such as the advocacy of a planning team in each district HA. For the most part, however, the recommendations in these parts of the report were either of a general hortatory kind (for example, everybody should be encouraged to try to get newly born babies registered with a GP, hotels should be encouraged to approach FPCs on the availability of local GPs), or couched in basic practical terms (for example, each health authority should be responsible for providing services to hotels in its area). It is in these parts of the report in particular that one gets the impression that the committee itself was unwilling to commit itself to priorities. The question 'which of these various recommendations would be most likely to improve primary health care in inner London?' is not answered by the committee and can only be guessed at by the reader. This is in contrast to the discussion of general practitioner services which, mainly because it is so much fuller and more sustained, does allow one to judge the relative importance of different parts of the argument.

Inner cities: cost of proposals
The importance of the question of priorities will be seen later in assessing the reaction to the Acheson report and measures which have been taken in response to it. Two other questions, on which the committee said little or nothing, also have a distinct bearing on the post-Acheson period. One is how far the Acheson analysis and recommendations are relevant only to London; the other is the cost of the proposals.

In describing the background to the appointment of the Acheson committee it was noted that concern with the difficulties of providing primary health care in the inner cities generally was one factor of particular importance in relating that appointment to its wider context. The terms of reference required the committee to consider only the situation in inner London, and apart from a brief reference to the fact that its recommendations might be applicable to other inner city areas[28], that is precisely what it did. Even where it drew comparisons between the structure of general practice in London and elsewhere, those comparisons were between inner and outer London and England and Wales as a whole[29]. It did not draw on such information as there was about other inner cities, such as the proportion of elderly doctors or of doctors not in group practice.

This was a strictly correct attitude, and certainly the committee would have been open to criticism if it had made pronouncements about the position in Birmingham or Manchester without having taken any evidence on it. Yet, as was suggested earlier, there was an ambiguity in the way the committee had been restricted to an examination of London problems but could not help being drawn into the consideration of wider issues, not least those affecting other inner cities. And although the report does not explicitly discuss general inner city issues, in other ways the committee showed its awareness of the fact that London problems could not be entirely resolved by measures applying only to London. Some recommendations required changes in national policies, especially those in connection with the retirement of GPs, where the committee was compelled to justify its recommendations in national rather than purely London terms. Thus in two rather different ways the Acheson report had relevance beyond London, explicitly in the way in which it discussed national policies, and implicitly in that it might be interpreted as having significance for other inner cities.

On the second question raised above, it is noteworthy that nowhere in the report is there any indication of how much the committee's proposals would cost. The brief reference to financial considerations is one of its least satisfactory parts. Recognising that there would be 'considerable resource consequences', i.e. that its proposals would cost a lot of money, it nevertheless relied on general arguments about the need to shift resources from acute hospital services to community services and primary care in London and indeed nationally as the main lever for achieving the objective of increased resources for primary health care. Claiming that the strategy for shifting resources in this way had been proposed by the LAG and endorsed by Ministers, it argued:

> the message is clear; resources *must* be redirected to community services if the strategy which has been adopted is to succeed. We do not presume that this redirection will be easily achieved—far from it—but we do presume that it will have the support of authorities and of Ministers[30].

These were bold words, but had the committee any real expectations that such a shift in resources was likely, and, if it had, why did it not also take the bolder step of trying to estimate what in fact its proposals would cost? Many, perhaps most, members of the committee would be inclined to say now that it was not so much realistic expectation as the need to deploy the only argument available to the committee. On the other hand, given the fact that there was a certain ambiguity when the committee was set up over the extent to which resources were likely to be made available for the improvement of primary health care in inner cities, it was perhaps not unreasonable to assume that, in the immediate context of the link between the Acheson inquiry and the proposals for reducing the number of acute beds in hospitals in inner London, sensible and workable proposals stood a good chance of being supported financially. During the course of the inquiry, however, as the committee put together a set of measures whose cost was not negligible, the government's drive to control and reduce public expenditure strengthened. Certainly, there must have been some doubt about the strength of Ministers' commitment to the LAG strategy of switching resources to primary health care for anyone reading Mr Patrick Jenkin's foreword to the LAG's report on acute hospital services. It is true that he gave general endorsement to the strategy, but specifically on the question of switching the resources saved on acute hospital services to other services he seemed to be offering a warning against over-optimism:

I agree with the thinking which has lead (sic!) to this conclusion. Of course, how resources are allocated nationally in future will depend on the determination of relative need in the Thames Regions and the rest of the country; and decisions will fall to be made at the time, in the light of the resources then available. But it would be misleading to assume that the kind of reductions here envisaged will of themselves always release disposable and therefore transferable resources. In many cases this will not be so; the staff and the buildings will continue to serve the community in other ways[31].

Of course, there were in any case considerable difficulties for the committee if it had wished to go further. There were, for example, practical difficulties in making realistic estimates of what its proposals would cost. But a more daunting difficulty one suspects was that too precise an assessment of costs would draw attention to the fact that London's gain might well be other areas' loss and would thus incur greater opposition to the proposals. The point here is that many proposals would cost little or nothing but only on the assumption that they were introduced within existing budgets, that is, by a switch of existing resources; if, for example, nurses were to be provided with extra support in the way of transport, clerical support etc., then this would either be at the expense of other items in the health authorities' budgets, or possibly at the expense of other health authorities' budgets (if other areas of the country were to receive less in order to meet London's needs); or it would have to be 'new money'.

The dilemma was most acute for the general practitioner services where the most expensive of the committee's proposals arose. Here it could be argued that the cost of some proposals would be balanced by savings on others. The proposals for initial group practice allowances, for example, would be more than balanced by savings on the level at which reductions in the basic practice allowance were introduced[32]. But the effect would be that some doctors would lose part of the allowances they were currently receiving and might therefore be expected to oppose the proposal. Similarly, a London weighting[33] was unlikely to receive much support outside London if its cost had to be borne effectively by doctors in the rest of the country. The really expensive item here was, however, the cost of compensation to elderly doctors on retirement. It was true that this would only be a temporary cost and that there might in the long run be some saving from reducing the number of elderly single-handed doctors, but here 'new money' was essential if the proposal was to be a success.

It is therefore easy to see the attraction for the committee in not going too closely into the financial implications of its proposals, and in suggesting that everything could be done by simply switching the resources saved on the acute hospital services to the primary sector. In that way new money could be represented as in effect old money, however difficult in practice, as the commitee realised, the actual process might prove; and the controversy and opposition which some of its proposals were bound to meet would at least not be exacerbated by making too precise who might be the losers financially. The danger was that the committee might be accused of lack of realism, whether in proposing expensive measures with no indication of cost or in relying on an uncertain idea that a rational switch of resources within the NHS could be carried out in practice.

Summing up

The main characteristics of the committee's work may be summed up as follows:

   i) *general approach*: a search for solutions within the framework of the existing system and in the light of generally held assumptions about the best way to organise primary health care;

   ii) *evidence*: although, as the report itself notes, there was wide agreement on the nature of the problems, the evidence was inconclusive on the measures needed to deal with them, and therefore left the committee to thrash out its own solution;

   iii) *recommendations*: a large number of recommendations was included in each area of discussion and analysis, ranging from major policy questions to relatively minor matters of procedure;

   iv) *priorities*: priorities were not indicated, whether through inability to agree, or through belief that it would not be meaningful to do so or possibly both;

   v) *short-term or long-term view*: again, the report did not restrict itself to short-term measures, and many of the most important recommendations were of a long-term nature.

The Acheson committee produced a solid well argued report whose convincingness nevertheless depended on acceptance of certain basic assumptions, for example, about the desirable way of organising primary health care. But those assumptions and indeed much of the analysis and many of the proposals put forward in the report were, one might say, part of the conventional wisdom to be found in much of the literature on primary health care in inner cities. That is not to detract from what the committee did. For one thing, its analysis and proposals were based on a much wider examination than any previous inquiry. The strong point of the report is above all its comprehensiveness[34]. It was the first time that the problems of primary health care in inner London, or indeed any inner city area, had been looked at comprehensively in this way, not only drawing widely on the existing literature but also searching out the views of those closely concerned with the provision of services.

To say that the report is well argued is not of course to say that some of the arguments are not open to criticism. Like all proponents of a case, the committee sometimes overstated its case[35]. In other ways, however, the report is remarkably open: on the need for more information on such subjects as the overlap between different medical practices or levels of staffing for nurses[36]; on the need for experimentation, for example, in the use of salaried assistants to general practitioners or devising a screening system for elderly patients[37]; and in its awareness that not all parts of inner London have the same problems and that therefore recommendations might need to be adapted to local circumstances[38].

This comprehensiveness and the anxiety to make sure that any views and ideas which might be relevant were brought to light and considered, which lay behind the committee's extensive seeking of evidence, was, however, achieved at a price. For those wanting a mine from which to quarry useful pieces the Acheson report is ideal. There they are—pieces on incentives for group practice, or making conditions for nurses more attractive, or the many other matters discussed in the report.

But policy makers might well wonder, where do we go from here? It is true that there is something for everybody in the report, but where should one begin, what would be the most useful starting point, what offers the best value for money if not everything can be done at once—or at all? On these questions the report offered little guidance. There was much in it for those who were anxious to make progress, but what sort of impact was it likely to have on the sceptical, those with no great interest in primary health care or those who were simply caught up in many other pressing problems of current concern?

Luck undoubtedly plays a part and often a large part in determining how far reports of committees of inquiry are implemented[39]. The right report must come at the right time. The government took no action on the Acheson report for two and a half years and the limited measures it then introduced related to primary health care in the inner cities generally and not just London. Was it the wrong report then, or did it arrive at the wrong time—or both? The next chapter will try to elucidate this question against the background of changing political and economic events.

References

1   For brevity, referred to simply as 'the committee'.
2   He was, for example, appointed to the University Grants Committee in 1981 and made chairman of its Medical Subcommittee.
3   See *Primary Health Care in Inner London : report of a study group*, LHPC, May 1981 (henceforth referred to as 'Report'), para 1.1.
4   Report, Annex 2.
5   Mr Patrick Jenkin in a debate on the National Health Service, HC Deb. 23 January 1980, vol. 977, col. 466.
6   Dr Gerard Vaughan, *ibid.*, cols 575-6; in his eagerness to stress the point he said that Acheson would be reporting in a few weeks!
7   On report stage of the Health Services Bill, HC Deb. 9 June 1980, vol. 986, cols 180-1: cf. HC Deb. 2 May 1980, vol. 983, WA 720.
8   *Report of Royal Commission on the National Health Service*, Cmnd 7615, HMSO, July 1979, para 7.63.
9   *Health Care in Big Cities*, International Hospital Federation, 1976.
10   Dr Brian Jarman, who was mainly responsible for carrying out the RCGP analysis, was a member of the Acheson committee; in September 1980 Margaret Lally, research assistant on the RCGP inquiry, was also appointed to the committee; she was by then working for the GLC.
11   See 'The family doctor in Central London', *Jl. RCGP,* October 1978, pp.606-17.
12   Report, para.1.11.
13   The area was not restricted to inner London but took in the whole of Greater London so that, for example, evidence was received from Barnet as well as Camden and Islington AHAs, from Hillingdon as well as City and East London FPCs.
14   A cheap reproduction process helped to cut down the time involved in the actual process of publication.

[15] For example, alternative arrangements involving the employment by health authorities of medical and other staff in clinics should be considered where conventional arrangements were failing to meet health care needs (Report, paras 4.69, 4.73). Health authorities were also encouraged to employ GPs on a sessional basis in accident and emergency departments as an experiment (para. 9.23).

[16] See his article 'Medical problems in Inner London', *Jl. RCGP*, October 1978, pp.598-602 and also the RCGP's *Survey of Primary Care in London*, 1981; he has also taken an active part in more recent attempts to identify underprivileged areas (see his articles in the *BMJ* on this, 28 May 1983, pp.1705-9 and 8 December 1984, pp.1587-92: also J.R.H. Charlton and Azim Lakhani, 'Is the Jarman underprivileged area score valid?' *BMJ*, 8 June 1985).

[17] For example, the BMA evidence began with a quotation from Michael Downham's article 'Medical care in inner cities', *BMJ*, 19 August 1978, p.545, 'Health services do not in the long term hold the key to the health and happiness of those living with the problems of our urban society. . .'

[18] Report, paras 3.2, 3.6.

[19] *Ibid.*, 3.7: and Margaret Bone, *Registration with General Medical Practitioners in Inner London*, HMSO, 1984.

[20] *A Survey of Primary Care in London*, RCGP, 1981, T.13.7: Report, T.5,p.21.

[21] For example, Professor David Morrell of St Thomas's Medical School, who gave evidence to the committee, had carried out a survey in his area which drew attention to the isolation in which many GPs worked (see D. Morrell, 'Inner London general practice: is there a solution?' *BMJ*, 10 January 1981, p.162).

[22] Report, paras 4.4, 4.6.

[23] *Ibid.*, paras 4.7, 4.8

[24] cf. 'The family doctor in Central London', *Jl. RCGP*, October 1978, p.607. As noted earlier, this was the report of a survey by Kensington, Chelsea and Westminster (South) CHC.

[25] Report, para. 4.19.

[26] The whole question of accessibility of GPs was clearly regarded as of considerable importance by the committee. Apart from examining the use of deputising services it commissioned a survey of telephone answering services, and found that the problem of answering machines was at least as great as that of the use of deputising services and indeed the two were often confused by members of the public (Report, paras. 3.18-22).

[27] See Jane Hughes and Jenny Roberts, 'Problems in the Development of London's Community Nursing Services', King's Fund Project Paper, *London's Health Services in the 80s*, No. 25, Pt. 3, April 1980.

[28] Report, para. 1.9.

[29] For example, Tables 3, 4 and 5.

[30] Report, para. 1.14.

[31] *Acute Hospital Services in London*, Report to the Secretary of State for Social Services by the London Advisory Group, January 1981, Foreword, para. 5.

[32] Report, paras. 4.21 and 4.25.

[33] *Ibid.*, para. 4.26.

[34] Even so, it had to leave out such important aspects as the dental and pharmaceutical services (Report, para 1.3).

[35] For example, it is by no means clear that if a retirement policy were brought in and if it created at least 40 vacancies, as the committee hoped, 'concerted action to provide a better framework within which the new GPs would work' would follow. (Report para 4.6).

[36] Report, paras 5.15, 6.25.

[37] *Ibid.*, paras 4.15, 7.24.

[38] *Ibid.*, para 1.18.

[39] Perhaps the most celebrated case of recent years is the Redcliffe Maud Commission on Local Government in England; having had their report largely accepted by the Labour government, they saw it rejected by the incoming Heath government in 1970.

CHAPTER 3   GOVERNMENT RESPONSE TO THE ACHESON REPORT

Introduction

This chapter deals essentially with the government's policy response to the report of the Acheson committee. The report contained a large number of recommendations, many of which were directed primarily at the numerous bodies with responsibilities in the primary care field, including regional and district health authorities, FPCs and local authorities. The next chapter will deal with the ways in which those bodies have responded to the ideas as well as the specific recommendations in the report. Government response can be considered in two ways: i) what encouragement it gave to other authorities to take up recommendations directed at them; ii) how it handled those parts of the report which required specific action by central government.

One preliminary point is that there were particular difficulties in the nature of the report. It is no doubt generally true that reports of committees of inquiry frequently reveal differences of attitude between the signatories of the report and the civil servants who have, within whatever political constraints currently apply, to decide what to do with it. What on one side appears as a coherent set of proposals in which the various aspects reinforce one another is likely to be dissected by the other to find what is possible and what impossible, what can be done fairly easily and what is likely to be troublesome to achieve. The Acheson report was the kind of report to make civil servants groan. Irrespective of the value of individual recommendations or groups of recommendations, its 'something for everybody' appearance made it difficult to know where to concentrate efforts. This is a factor to be taken into account when considering the reception of the report against the political and economic background of the early 1980s.

A further preliminary point is that the Harding report was published on the same day as the Acheson report. Many of its recommendations were of a general nature, but one chapter was devoted to problems specific to particular geographical areas, especially the inner cities. On the whole, the Harding analysis reinforced that of the Acheson report and, indeed, what the Royal Commission had said earlier on the provision of primary health care in declining urban areas, but it laid particular emphasis on the difficulties of applying the team concept in inner city areas. Many of the Harding recommendations were on similar lines to those of Acheson, but understandably they could not pursue in detail questions which loomed large for Acheson, such as the need to encourage elderly GPs with small lists to retire. Although the Harding report will not be considered in detail here, it is worth noting that the government tended to link it with the Acheson report, partly no doubt for tactical reasons in attempting to answer charges of slowness in making a response by pointing out that to the 115 recommendations which had to be considered from the Acheson committee there had to be added another 50 from the Harding committee[1].

There is a final preliminary point here. Formally, the Acheson committee made its report to the LHPC which had appointed it in the first place. This was indeed a formality and effectively the report was made to the Secretary of State. Shortly after the Acheson report was published, the LHPC ceased to exist. Since that time there has been no formal machinery for dealing with London health problems embracing all the various authorities with responsibilities in the field. Symbolically, therefore, 1981 marks the end of one of those periodic phases when London problems seem to surface and compel attention.

When the Acheson committee reported there was, however, one other temporary body which had to be brought into the reckoning. The London Advisory Group's scrutiny of the report formed part of its final report which was published in the same month, May 1981, after which the LAG too ceased to exist.

The LAG's main contribution, so far as primary care is concerned, was to argue strongly for the diversion of resources saved on acute hospital services to primary health care, and to press for urgent action by central government to strengthen primary health care in London. These themes had formed a prominent part of the LAG's earlier report on the hospital services[2]. They were reinforced in the final report. Not only did the LAG's strategy for the acute hospital services depend:

> fundamentally for its success on a complementary strengthening of the primary health care services

but it was vital that an overall thrust towards the agreement and implementation of the necessary changes should be maintained from the centre since only the Department:

> is in a position to ensure that concerted action is taken by all the responsible authorities.

In his covering letter Sir John Habbakuk went further in a personal appeal to Mr Jenkin:

> we are greatly concerned that without your personal commitment to effecting the sort of changes proposed, little progress will be made in this vital area[3].

The message was clear. Act urgently and forcefully and provide the resources to make action effective. In one sense this could be seen as doing no more than taking up what Ministers themselves had been saying at the time when the Acheson committee was set up[4]. Had they not stressed the need for rapid and effective action? Here, then, in the primary care field was the opportunity. But were the Acheson recommendations quite what they had in mind? And how far, when it came to the point, were they prepared to make a commitment, and especially a financial commitment, to the improvement of London's primary health care services?

Certainly, the RHAs, AHAs and FPCs in London were told when the Acheson report was published that Ministers welcomed it and they were asked to 'give it urgent consideration as a basis for action'. Copies of the report and this message were also sent not only to local authorities, the University of London, CHCs and LMCs, but also to all GPs in London and everybody who had given evidence to the committee. All were invited to comment on the report. At the same time, the Department was said to be considering recommendations which were its responsibility. The Minister of State did, however, refer to the argument that the money saved on reducing the number of acute hospital beds could be used to build up the primary care services:

> I am sure that this is the way to get a better medical service for the people of London[5].

On the face of it, then, the initial reaction from government was reasonably encouraging to the Acheson committee. It went a little further than is the case with most committees of inquiry in actually commending the report for action to the various health authorities. On the other hand, as Rudolf Klein has pointed out, for effective and successful implementation of national priorities in the NHS there needs to be 'continued pressure and intervention' by the DHSS[6], and there is no evidence that the Department intended to follow up its original commendation of the report. Indeed, when the government was later criticised for inaction over the Acheson report it pointed to the fact that many of the recommendations were directed at other bodies rather than central government and that these bodies had been asked to consider action on them as an indication of the government's concern with and acceptance of 'the broad thrust' of the Acheson report[7]. Of course, one may argue that at that stage, over a year after the Acheson report had appeared, the government was very much on the defensive over its failure to make any specific response to the report, and therefore naturally made the most of the fact that many of the report's recommendations were not specifically directed at it. The point to be made here, however, is that even in these circumstances there was no suggestion of anything more being done than commending the report to other authorities and, in effect, leaving it to them to decide whether to take action or not.

Factors affecting initial reaction: finding the money; London or all inner cities; persistence of inner city health care issue
Inevitably, however, the main discussion here must relate to the parts of the Acheson report which required a positive response from central government if

effective action was to be taken on them. That initial government reaction was fairly non-committal is not surprising. On most committee reports governments invite comments and have discussions with the various interests concerned before either announcing specific proposals or simply taking no further action. It only becomes surprising when set against ministerial pronouncements in 1980 which stressed the need for urgent action. The discrepancy became even more pronounced when government response to the Acheson report suffered a series of postponements.

One clue to the discrepancy is to be found in the ambiguity of motive in setting up the Acheson inquiry in the first place which was commented on in the previous chapter. By the time the committee reported in 1981 ministerial expectations had moved more definitely in the direction of a limited report in both time and scope and, therefore, most importantly, a report likely to cost relatively little to implement. What the committee had provided, however, was an extensive report with numerous recommendations and 'considerable resource consequences'.

At first sight, the argument that resources saved from reductions in the acute hospital sector could be diverted into the primary sector seemed to provide a possible means of reconciling the two approaches. Unfortunately, the practical application of this idea raises all manner of difficulties. To begin with, it was not simply a question of reducing the number of acute beds in inner London, but of the distribution of such beds throughout the area of the four Thames regions. Inner London was over-provided with beds but to some extent this was balanced by under-provision elsewhere in the regions. The LHPC's assessment, although carefully qualified, makes this clear. Scarcely any inner London area was thought to need additional beds, whereas many areas beyond Greater London did. Since, however, the numbers of the latter were mainly fairly modest compared with some drastic reductions within London, the net effect was a reduction in beds for all four regions between 1977 and 1988, amounting in total to about 10 per cent of the numbers in 1977[8].

This apparent scope for savings has to be set in a wider context. Under the national RAWP formula each of the four Thames regions was to have a reduced share of total NHS allocations. In the later 1970s and early 1980s there was little or no real growth in NHS expenditure, with the consequence that competition for funds within regional budgets grew more intense, and most intense of all in the Thames regions which in some years had their budgets reduced in real terms[9].

To this must be added the warning given by Mr Jenkin that in purely physical terms the savings on acute hospital beds might not be readily convertible into transferable resources[10]. Indeed, an analysis made by two writers in the *British Medical Journal* using the admittedly limited data available reached the tentative conclusion:

that appreciable savings will not accrue in real terms[11].

Given this situation, there are obvious difficulties in achieving any significant switch of resources from hospital to primary care services in the regions and districts. Moreover, a change of priorities of this kind can always be done more easily if additional funds are available, a situation unlikely to arise in present circumstances.

A further obstacle is the separate financing arrangements for the family practitioner services. These depend not on the determination of a total sum to be distributed to individual FPCs but on demand for the services. As the DHSS has acknowledged, the system poses formidable difficulties for both forecasting and controlling expenditure. Even if a precise figure of savings in the hospital sector could be determined, there is no way in which this could be directly made available to the FPS. There are of course ways in which the Department can influence both the amount of money going to these services and, equally important, the direction in which it goes. The recent proposal for a limited list of drugs for prescribing is one obvious example.

More relevant here is the fact that the method of determining the remuneration of general practitioners makes it possible to provide incentives to promote particular purposes of policy, and of course some of the Acheson recommendations were of this nature, but, as is discussed later, this raises other difficulties about the consequential effects of introducing incentives of this kind.

A further difficulty of a quite different kind affected this question of diverting resources into primary health care. Although the whole raison d'etre of the Acheson inquiry as it emerged from the LHPC/LAG mechanism was to deal with difficulties which had their origins in specifically London circumstances, that justification became progressively less persuasive as attention moved away from the problem of acute beds in hospital to that of primary health care. The reason is simply that whereas in the acute sector the major problems were mainly, if not exclusively, due to developments peculiar to London, this was not the case with primary health care. Any study of primary health care in London could not be restricted simply to those aspects which were unique to London but would inevitably deal with matters which affected to a greater or lesser degree other areas of the country, and especially other inner city areas.

Furthermore, it must have been clear when the Acheson report was published—or if it was not the GMSC must soon have made it clear—that in matters affecting general practitioners the profession was most unlikely to be willing to accept measures which applied only to London practitioners, particularly, it should be added, if the cost of such measures were to fall effectively on other GPs[12]. The history of attempts within the profession to secure a London weighting for GPs provides a locus classicus for this kind of approach. At LMC annual conferences and meetings of the GMSC the question of a London weighting was raised from time to time. But even when motions were specifically worded to make it clear that it would only be acceptable if 'new money' was available to finance it, so that the cost would not be met by reducing the money available for other doctors, they were always defeated by arguments as various as that other areas also experienced an above-average cost of living or that in others such as South Wales the life of a GP was harder than in London.

The nearest the movers of such motions came to success was when they widened the scope to metropolitan areas generally and not just London[13].

The significance of the profession's attitude was that it raised the question whether, if the Acheson report's recommendations were to be taken up, it should not be on a broader front. The most obvious approach would be to consider proposals applying to inner cities generally. The immediate consequence would be to increase the cost of implementing the Acheson proposals if they were to be applied to all inner cities. That at least would be true of those proposals applying to GPs which had a specific area application like increased improvement grants or additional incentives to group practice. Some of the other proposals, as the Acheson report acknowledged, would in any case need to be introduced nationally, notably retirement policy for GPs, and could not just apply to London or even the inner cities generally. Nevertheless, the extension of the Acheson proposals to all inner city areas could not fail to make some increase in the cost of implementation inevitable.

The second main point, however, about extending the Acheson proposals is that to do so would diminish, if not destroy, the rational basis of the Acheson and LAG view that improvement in primary health care could be brought about by re-directing resources from the hospital sector, simply because, as has been said, over-provision of acute hospital beds was mainly a London phenomenon.

The conclusion seems inescapable that whatever Acheson and LAG might argue, and whatever indeed Dr Vaughan's immediate reaction might be, any money which was needed to implement the Acheson proposals would have to be specially provided. Even if the specific amounts saved by the bed closure programme in London could be precisely identified and an equivalent amount provided for primary health care, this would in practice be 'new money'. And if the approach were changed to the improvement of primary health care in the inner cities generally, then this would be still more obviously the case.

But how much money was involved? It is difficult to give a precise answer. Acheson did not do the sums and nobody since has attempted to publish any precise figures. Yet the question is important not only for its effect on what was done or not done in response to Acheson but for assessing how adequate was the money eventually provided by the government in relation to the needs of primary health care in the inner cities.

Shortly after the committee reported Professor Acheson was quoted as saying that he thought a lot could be done for £5m[14]. That was presumably for inner London alone, and the amount would have to be doubled or more to cover all the inner cities. A further difficulty is that recurring payments have to be separated from once-for-all expenditure. Increased improvement grants might cost a good deal initially but would then tail off once premises had been improved; registration fees and central funding of nurse training would represent continuing costs. Most items on the Acheson list were difficult to cost precisely. Improvement grants provide an example. How many doctors would apply and what the cost of improvements would be and which grants would be claimed were speculative questions. The additional cost of improvement grants if about half the inner London doctors applied for them and the average cost of improvements was £30,000 would be about £5m[15], but if fewer doctors applied and the cost of improvements was less this figure might be halved[16].

One can appreciate the difficulties the Acheson committee would have had in making meaningful estimates of cost, and yet something could have been done. In 1981 terms perhaps £5.10m would have covered the initial costs, with then a recurring £1.2m per annum. That is for London alone. For the inner cities as a whole one might suggest £15.25m with a recurring £2.5m per annum. Imprecise sums, but very much in line with the 'off the cuff' approach which was all the chairman of the GMSC could offer[17]. More important here than the actual sums is the fact that they were comparatively small in relation to the total expenditure on primary health care services. In 1981/82 current expenditure on the family practitioner services amounted to £2,440m, to which must be added a comparatively small part of the £7,631m spent on the hospital and community health services. Even if the whole of the initial cost of the Acheson proposals had fallen in one year, it would have represented less than an additional one per cent of expenditure. In practice the cost would have been spread over several years. Continuing costs would have been very much less.

In addition, there were some savings or potential savings in the Acheson proposals which could be set against the total gross cost. The most obvious savings derived from the suggestion that the threshold for payment of the full basic practice allowance and certain other payments should be raised from 1000 patients on a list to 1500. However reasonable that might appear, it was obviously going to be a difficult matter to negotiate since it would mean that some doctors would lose part of the income to which they had previously been entitled. Among potential savings would again be savings on the basic practice allowance if the Acheson proposals for reducing the number of elderly single-handed doctors with small lists achieved their aim. Potential savings, however, have a habit of not materialising, or certainly not as fully as optimistic advocates claim, whereas expenditure which incidentally may promote the savings is all too real.

It has been necessary to deal at some length with the question of the cost of the Acheson proposals and its implications simply because it was obviously going to be one main issue. It was not, however, necessarily the most important issue and certainly not the only one which was likely to affect the response the government would make to the Acheson report. In a sense, financial considerations were only one part of a much wider problem for the government, which was how to make a response which would show that it was doing something about the problems without becoming involved in what might well turn out to be undesirable long-term commitments. That this was seen as a dilemma is perhaps implicit in the fact that a long period elapsed between publication of the Acheson report in May 1981 and the detailed government response of October 1983.

On the one side, there was the inescapable fact of the continuing existence of difficulties in providing adequate primary health care services in the inner cities, and pressure from the medical profession for action to be taken to remedy the situation. Ironically, the Acheson report reinforced this pressure in spite of the fact that it had seemed to be concerned only with a much more limited aspect. But the depth of the committee's analysis, even though it was confined to one particular inner city area, made much more explicit the nature of the problems faced in the inner cities and thus provided a clearer focus on them. Against this, the government had to decide how much priority to give to primary health care in the inner cities.

In other words, the implication of the Acheson analysis was that it was no longer sufficient to look to some limited measures to meet the immediate London problem. Some response would have to be made touching on the problems of providing primary health care in the inner cities generally, or else the government would have to reject Acheson entirely, as it had recently rejected the Black report.

That rejection might be seen as an indication of the Conservative government's tough line towards reports conceived by its predecessor, particularly those involving increased public expenditure. The Black report had advocated both a shift of resources within the NHS towards community care, and, more generally, a programme of public expenditure on a fairly large scale to make an impact on existing inequalities. The response of the Secretary of State, published as a foreword to the report only a few months before the Acheson report was published, left no doubt of the government's position:

> additional expenditure on the scale which could result from the report's recommendations . . . is quite unrealistic in present or any foreseeable economic circumstances . . . I cannot, therefore, endorse the Group's recommendations[18].

The cost of Acheson could not compare with the 'upwards of £2 billion a year' which Mr Jenkin suggested might result from the Black report's recommendations, nor was primary health care in London or the inner cities a subject as daunting and vast as the causes of inequality in health between social classes. Any temptation the government might have had to 'do a Black' on Acheson came up against the very different circumstances of the two reports. In spite of the unwelcome nature of some of the Acheson recommendations, the intractable problems of the inner cities in general and of primary health care in particular could not be ignored.

Furthermore, the review of the inner city policy of the Labour government, and in particular the partnership and programme authority arrangements which had been instituted in 1977, resulted in a continuation of the arrangements, although the scale of expenditure was to be less than that planned by the Labour government[19]. As in 1977 health matters did not figure prominently in the discussions, but the riots which broke out in Brixton and later in other inner city areas in the spring and summer of 1981 served to keep the inner cities on the policy agenda. That, and the fact, as has been pointed out earlier, that primary health care in the inner cities was a recurring theme in the health policy field ensured that government would be expected to make some response to the cry from the medical profession and elsewhere of crisis in primary care in inner cities. Indeed, some tangible acknowledgement of the problems had been made shortly before the Acheson committee reported. The DHSS had made a grant of £540,000 to the Department of General Practice of Manchester University to carry out research into inequalities of medical care in inner city areas[20].

The Acheson report could not therefore simply be ignored. On the other hand, it could not simply be accepted as it stood, if only because of the need to translate it into an inner city rather than a London document. The dilemma was perhaps particularly acute for the Minister with the main responsibility for making an initial response to the report, Dr Gerard Vaughan. A consultant at Guy's Hospital before becoming an MP, he probably did not regard solving the problems of primary health care in the inner cities as one of his urgent priorities. At all events, he gave the impression of someone treading carefully and not very enthusiastically into what must have seemed a political minefield, where the possibility of conflict with the professions and his own colleagues if he pressed too hard for the Acheson proposals had to be balanced against the pressure to do something about primary health care in the inner cities. Thus, at first the government appeared to be casting around for a solution which would enable it to claim that it was doing something about the problems without involving itself in too many troublesome questions.

The uncertainty of attitude is shown by the fact that towards the end of 1981 the King's Fund was approached for its suggestions on how best to improve primary health care in London if £1m or £2m was made available for this purpose[21]. This was perhaps the first indication of the approach which governed the months which followed the government's acknowledgement that it would have to commit some extra money to the inner cities but its reluctance to take the hard decisions on the exact measures to be supported.

Views of the professions

If there was thus a certain reluctance by the government to take up the Acheson recommendations, and then only in relation to inner cities generally, where else might the committee get support? The medical press reacted reasonably favourably to the report but with a certain scepticism about the likelihood of progress being made. Thus the *British Medical Journal* ended its account of the report with the words:

but the important question now is will anything happen?[22]

A writer in *The Lancet* argued more subtly that what lay behind both the Acheson and Harding reports was a plea for extra money for primary health care, but in existing economic circumstances that was most unlikely to be offered:

in which case primary care can be improved only at the expense of hospital care[23].

Clearly, some proposals attracted attention because they were controversial and the source of disagreements within the profession, and this was especially true of the retirement proposals, but the underlying uneasiness was whether the government was likely to be willing to provide the additional money which the bulk of the major recommendations required[24].

But it was not so much initial reaction as considered views which were most likely to influence the government. And here, although it was clearly important to know what view the health authorities, FPCs and such bodies as the Medical Practices Committee took of the Acheson report, the vital element was the reaction of the professions, and especially the medical profession in view of the large number of recommendations in the report which affected that profession.

Perhaps not surprisingly the Royal College of Nursing supported, and often strongly supported, practically the whole of the Acheson recommendations. The report did after all acknowledge that living and working conditions for nurses in inner London needed to be improved, and its major policy recommendations, such as that there should be central funding for nurse training or that establishments for nurses in inner London should be increased, were clearly welcome to the RCN as tending to strengthen the position of nurses working in inner London.

The position was somewhat more complicated so far as the medical profession was concerned since the GMSC not only had to comment on the report but was also the body which would negotiate with the government on those matters affecting the pay and conditions of service of GPs. A further complication was that the RCGP also had a considerable interest in the Acheson recommendations. There tended to be a rather uneasy relationship between the College and the GMSC ever since the former had been founded in the 1950s and had become the recognised voice of the profession in matters relating to professional education and training.

There was a curious contrast in the evidence presented to the Acheson committee by the two bodies. The GMSC's evidence presented through the BMA was rather low key, and tended to emphasise the need for more research into the state of primary health care in London. Among its positive suggestions, however, was the view that the remuneration of GPs might be modified along the lines of proposals made by the working group on under-privileged areas. The RCGP by contrast had provided the Acheson committee with a broader view of the problems, but had not spelled out in detail what might be done about them except in advocating the extension and strengthening of academic departments of general practice, which was of course part of its major concern. Nevertheless, it too advocated identifying deprived areas possibly on a population density basis and paying a special allowance to doctors practising there. It also made some general suggestions about the use of financial incentives, for example to encourage older doctors to retire.

There was thus an initial problem for the two bodies in deciding how they would respond to the Acheson report and in particular for which aspects of the report each should take primary responsibility. There already existed a liaison committee with members drawn from both bodies which met regularly to discuss matters of mutual concern, and it was to this forum that the question of who should make the primary response to the various recommendations was referred. In the event, there was a broad measure of agreement between them and differences were largely a matter of emphasis. In many cases indeed the RCGP was in the position of supporting measures which the GMSC was in favour of and had the main responsibility for, such as the payment of a registration fee for new patients. Both could also agree broadly on measures to improve practice premises or to promote the effective working of the primary health care team, even though they might not agree in detail on the measures to be taken[25].

In responding to the Acheson report the GMSC made two general points which are not unexpected in view of what has been said earlier: that many of the problems identified applied also in other inner city areas, and that the work of the GMSC's working group on under-privileged areas could be an important pointer to the way forward. Taken together these points added up to a decisive statement of the GMSC's position that any measures resulting from the Acheson report should be of general application and not specifically applied only to London. A clear hint was given that only on this basis was there likely to be agreement from the profession. A London weighting for GPs was therefore rejected by the GMSC, whereas, for example, proposals for minimum standards for premises and routine visiting of premises by FPCs were acceptable provided that they applied nationally. On the other hand, the GMSC found the idea of paying salaries to GPs anathema even in the very limited guise suggested by Acheson of an experimental scheme of salaried assistants in single-handed practices where the principal was near retirement.

But perhaps the most crucial set of recommendations for the profession were those related to Acheson's central theme of the need to reduce the number of elderly single-handed doctors, especially those with small lists, and to attract young doctors to work in inner London with, it was hoped, a greater commitment to group practice and working in a primary care team. There was a dilemma here, particularly recognised by the RCGP. Single-handed doctors could not be condemned as a whole but, on the other hand, too many single-handed doctors with small lists made it difficult to achieve the aim which the College fully endorsed of providing primary health care largely through teams. It therefore supported the Acheson retirement and associated superannuation proposals on the grounds that these only affected elderly doctors who might otherwise have to continue working because they could not afford to retire.

For the GMSC, on the other hand, it was precisely the idea of compelling GPs to retire which was the main stumbling block in the Acheson proposals, mainly because it was acutely sensitive to the need to preserve the 'independent contractor' status of GPs which had become an article of faith of the BMA, and retirement policy could be seen as detracting from that status, the 'thin end of the wedge' which might lead to further central determination of the conditions of service of GPs. Nevertheless, the Acheson proposals had served to put retirement policy for GPs back on the agenda. The response of the GMSC was predictable; it was against compulsory retirement but in favour of inducements to retire, such as more favourable pension arrangements for elderly GPs, on the same grounds as the RCGP's response that it was undesirable that GPs should have to carry on working because they could not afford to retire. This approach, reliance on the carrot rather than the stick, fell a good deal short of what Acheson had intended. For a major aim of the committee had been to create a comparatively large number of vacancies within a short space of time, and it was very uncertain what effect inducements to retire voluntarily would have, particularly in view of the results of Acheson's own survey of elderly doctors, which showed that most of them went on working because they wanted to and not because they had to for financial reasons[26].

There were other aspects of the Acheson report which the GMSC did not like, such as its strictures on the inadequacy of some GPs' telephone answering arrangements[27] and its view that the arrangements for deputising services should be tightened up. Aside from these sensitive areas and major policy issues like retirement and payment of salaries, the GMSC generally supported the Acheson report, not only on such matters as the provision of bigger improvement grants for improvement of premises and payment of an additional fee for new patients where one might have expected its support, but also on organisational matters such as the establishment of management units for community services in health districts and of primary health care planning teams. It was also in favour of the 'facilitator' idea, that is, someone specifically charged with offering advice and assistance to GPs, particularly in connection with premises and facilities. Where, however, the Acheson recommendations were likely to affect some existing GPs adversely, especially from a financial point of view, there was again opposition from the GMSC. The most obvious example was the proposal to raise the size of list for the payment of full practice expenses, but it is also noticeable that the GMSC was not in favour of the DHSS issuing guidelines to the MPC and FPCs, the effect of which would be to encourage the appointment of young and therefore less experienced GPs to inner city practices.

The RCGP, in accordance with the agreed division of responsibilities with the GMSC, gave more general support to many of these ideas, such as the need to promote improvements in GPs' premises. Its main points were in the support of strengthened departments of general practice in the medical schools, and in developing the idea of facilitators. Here it wanted not only a medical adviser with broader functions in each region, but also an adviser in each district with particular responsibilities in the field of education of general practitioners.

The message therefore from the professions to the DHSS was clearly that they wanted something done to improve primary health care in the inner cities and that the Acheson report could at least be the starting point of measures to be taken to this end. It was, nevertheless, perfectly obvious to everybody that many of the measures which had most support would cost money. Indeed, in a sense one of the main attractions of the Acheson report to the professions was that it made clear both the nature of the measures which needed to be taken and the fact that money would have to be channelled into primary health care in the inner cities if there was to be any hope of those measures succeeding. As always, the critical question was where the money was to come from. For the GMSC it was clearly not to come from reductions in the amounts going to other GPs nor even from savings on other parts of the NHS. Its explicit view was that to be effective any response from the government would require the commitment of additional financial resources.

Difficulties and delays in government response

Financial considerations, as has been suggested, were important for the DHSS but they were not the only factors to be taken into account. No doubt they are the main reason why some Acheson proposals, although supported by the professions, have not been heard of again, such as the suggestion of paying an additional sum to GPs for each new patient. Even here, however, it was not just the cost but the likely consequences of proposals which had to be assessed. Could the cost be justified in terms of the likely effect on the number of people getting on to doctors' lists? With other proposals there might be doubt about their effectiveness: whether, for example, even if money was available, initial group practice allowances were the most effective means of encouraging group practice. Nevertheless, following the receipt of responses from the professional bodies, the DHSS opened formal discussions in the winter of 1981/82. The GMSC later claimed that by early 1982 certain 'understandings' had been reached with the DHSS on some Acheson issues[28]. The discussions were serious and wide-ranging, reflecting the view on both sides that some initiatives had to be taken on primary care in inner cities. Among the issues discussed at length, some were difficult and contentious, including retirement for GPs.

Yet it was not until November 1982 that the government announced in general terms some special support for primary health care in the inner cities, and not until October of the following year that a more specific announcement of a three-year programme was made. The long delay led to much speculative comment in the medical press, some of it contradictory. It is indeed not possible to be precise about the various manoeuvres and discussions which went on behind the scenes during this period. Various factors may have contributed to the delay. Politically, changes in the ministerial team may have been one. In September 1981 Mr Norman Fowler succeeded Mr Jenkin as Secretary of State and in the following April Dr Vaughan was replaced as Minister of State by Mr Kenneth Clarke, so that what some of the medical press liked to refer to as 'the ministerial double act' was completely changed[29].

It seems likely, however, that the main practical difficulties were over how much money could be found for improving primary health care in inner cities, and over devising an acceptable scheme for encouraging elderly doctors to retire. The two were, of course, connected since cost was a major factor in any retirement plan. Some of the medical press were confidently predicting in December 1981 a 'multi million pound package' for the inner cities by Easter 1982[30]. What was actually announced in November 1982 was much less precise. An additional £20m was being made available for the NHS in 1983/84:

for central initiatives to support new pilot schemes to benefit particular services where we are determined to raise standards and which will benefit most from this approach.

Among the half dozen areas which would share this £20m, primary health care in inner cities was merely noted as one which was likely to benefit[31]. Later Mr Fowler was a little more explicit, saying that 'more than £3 million' was available for the development of primary health care in inner cities, and: 'the initiative is the result of our consideration of the Acheson report. . . and of the Harding report . . . Broadly, we accept the diagnoses made by Acheson and Harding on primary care in inner cities'[32].

It was, however, very much in keeping with the long-drawn-out saga of the government's response to the Acheson report that although the Secretary of State ended this second statement by saying that he hoped to announce detailed proposals, no such announcement was ever made, at least until the rather different statement of October 1983. In February 1983 Mr Kenneth Clarke said he intended to make a statement soon; in March he hoped to publish plans shortly; by the end of April he was saying that the delay was 'because of the work and discussion involved in finalising the proposals'; but as in 1982 the weeks passed and there was silence[33].

It seems clear then that at a fairly early stage, either in the winter of 1981/82 or in the following spring, the government had committed itself to doing something about primary health care in inner cities. By July 1982, when the Labour Opposition initiated a debate on health care in inner London, the government, although having nothing positive to offer, accepted:

> the broad thrust of the Acheson report and the need to put as many of its proposals as practical into operation[34].

There was thus a period of about eighteen months between commitment in principle and the announcement of specific measures. The November 1982 announcement, especially as it was not followed by any details[35], thus appears rather as a holding device while decisions still had to be made about the nature and scope of measures to be introduced. The government could not go on indefinitely saying that it was generally in favour of Acheson without making some more positive commitment to specific measures. To say that £3m was being made available at least showed some commitment, although the impact was lessened by the failure to provide any indication of how the money was to be spent.

Ministers had of course more immediate and troublesome preoccupations in relation to the NHS; in 1982, for example, there was the lengthy dispute over nurses' pay. In 1983, however, as a general election drew nearer, there would have been some political advantage for Mr Fowler, as a commentator in *The Lancet* pointed out, in making some response to those parts of the Acheson report which, unlike the retirement issue, did not involve long and difficult negotiations[36]. But, as always, financial difficulties were prominent. The question of imposing cash limits on FPS expenditure was raised and referred by the government to a firm of accountants (Binder Hamlyn). Their investigation was carried out at the end of 1982 and in the early part of 1983 and thus posed a question mark over possible initiatives on the Acheson report. Then again once the election was over the new Chancellor of the Exchequer (Mr Nigel Lawson) pressed for reductions in the current year's public expenditure, including £100m for the NHS, which again for a time became an immediate preoccupation leading to well publicised confrontations with leaders of the medical profession[37].

There were thus plenty of reasons unconnected with the Acheson report and negotiations on it which may have contributed to delay, but it is also worth considering two factors more directly related to Acheson and connected with the retirement issue. Much stress was laid by the government on the need for extensive consultation on the Harding and Acheson reports. It was indeed the only defence it could make in public when charged with having done nothing about the reports. At the time of the November 1982 announcement the suggestion was made that Ministers were anxious to see elderly GPs give up their practices in inner cities, and that the reason for the delay in announcing a response to Acheson was that they wanted the GMSC to commit itself to at least an acknowledgement in principle that it was desirable for GPs to retire at 70[38].

It is very likely that discussions between the DHSS and the GMSC over retirement proved among the more difficult of the post-Acheson negotiations, but it hardly seems likely that the desire to persuade the GMSC to go along with a retirement policy could have been a major factor in the delays. It is, of course, quite plausible that the DHSS should argue that if the GMSC wanted additional money for GPs retirement policy should form part of the bargain. But given the GMSC's stance on the retirement question, it must surely have soon become obvious that even a commitment of this nature would require long and difficult negotiations. Was it worth holding up the entire Acheson package for this, rather than concentrating on where agreement might be possible? There was, for example, plenty of scope for discussion on the nature of other inducements to retirement where the GMSC had indicated its agreement.

There was indeed one good reason why it would have made sense to try to secure agreement with the GMSC on retirement policy. If money was to be used to promote the departure of elderly GPs from inner cities, a better case could be made for the expenditure if it was linked with a general change of policy requiring GPs to retire at 70, as proposed by Acheson. As it was, the medical press was full of circumstantial rumours that a prolonged argument had taken place between the DHSS and the Treasury over the former's proposal to offer cash inducements to inner city GPs of 74 and over to retire. It was said that Treasury objections were three-fold: the proposal would be very expensive; it would create an undesirable precedent; and it would be difficult to define which doctors should qualify[39].

It is certainly plausible to suppose that the Treasury might jib at the cost of inducing elderly doctors to retire, although in the absence of the precise proposals made by the DHSS it is impossible to know just how costly they were. The Acheson committee said that there were 106 GPs in inner London over th' age of 70; if each of them were to have received £15,000, that amounted to just over £1m; adding in the remainder of the inner cities would have made it perhaps £3m. Probably the DHSS was thinking in terms of smaller sums and a later age of retirement. These are not, therefore, very large amounts of money, but one suspects that there may have been some scepticism about the use of such inducements, given the findings of the Acheson survey of elderly GPs showing that lack of money was not the main reason why they continued to practise.

Perhaps of more importance was Treasury resistance to what, as compared with expenditure on the hospital services, was seen as uncontrollable expenditure on the family practitioner services including the general medical services. The Social Services Committee recently pointed out that over the five years 1979/80 to 1984/85 the FPS have grown in real terms faster than the NHS as a whole[40]. But then the rest of the NHS is subject to cash limits, whereas no way has so far been found of applying cash limits to the FPS whose expenditure therefore continues to be largely determined by demand[41]. When the July 1983 cuts in public expenditure were made, they affected in the NHS mainly the hospital and community health services. It was widely believed that the cuts were made to compensate for overspending although DHSS officials later implied that it was coincidence that the £100m cut from the HCHS budget was the same amount as overspending then expected on the FPS[42]. In any case one can understand Treasury irritation at the inability to control expenditure on the FPS, and its consequent opposition to proposals to increase that expenditure.

The other main objection alleged to have been brought by the Treasury is at first sight more puzzling. In recent years inducements to leave public sector industries where a reduction in the labour force is regarded as desirable have become common, particularly in the steel and coal mining industries. One might therefore see a parallel in offering payments to GPs in inner cities as an inducement to cease practising, without creating an 'undesirable precedent'. There are two reasons why the parallel cannot be pursued. In the first place, the object is not so much to reduce the total number of GPs, although that might be the effect if elderly doctors with small lists were the main people to retire, but rather to replace one set of doctors with another. Secondly, and of more importance, retirement is not the same as redundancy. GPs had been free to join the NHS superannuation scheme since 1948 and were, therefore, already in theory provided for as far as retirement was concerned. As the Acheson survey showed, most elderly doctors in inner London had joined the scheme and were in fact drawing their NHS pensions[43]. It might be that because of the comparatively limited number of years of practice from 1948 until the age of 65 the pension was—or seemed to be—inadequate, particularly where NHS pre-retirement income had been comparatively low and expenses comparatively high, as was often the case in inner London. The doubt was, however, whether it was right to commit extra resources to making good a temporary defect in an
fectly good pension scheme simply in order to further other
ever desirable these might be.
iculties of this kind had arisen can be inferred from arguments

put by Mr Kenneth Clarke early in 1983 against the introduction of such financial inducements:

> it cannot be argued that everybody who retires from a particular profession over the age of 65 should necessarily be entitled to compensation. It is extremely difficult to enhance the superannuation rights of people in a particular profession because it is thought that some of them have not a sufficiently good superannuation agreement[44].

Here, then, was the 'undesirable precedent' argument, although it could have been claimed that the situation was unique since no one else in the public sector had the independent contractor status of GPs which was the root cause of difficulties. Nevertheless, there was clearly a distinction between doing what Acheson had recommended, that is, introducing a general policy of retirement at a certain age, for which corresponding financial arrangements could be made, and using financial inducements to deal with a temporary problem in London and perhaps other inner cities. The Acheson committee had quite clearly seen the problem, and, as has been shown, had attempted to justify a retirement policy on general grounds and not simply as a way of getting round the fact that there were too many elderly single-handed GPs in London. But once the idea of compulsory retirement was dropped, it was no longer possible to disguise the fact that financial inducements to retire were simply a means for dealing with the temporary problem.

A further point to be remembered here is that it was by no means clear what the effect of introducing financial inducements to retire would be. The aim, after all, was not just to get rid of elderly GPs but to bring in young doctors committed to group practice and the primary health care team concept. All the members of the Acheson committee except one believed that a retirement policy was a necessary condition of achieving this aim, but it was not sufficient in itself. Even if the modified plan to offer financial inducements created vacancies, how those vacancies were filled depended on the attitudes of FPCs and the MPC. There was no question of telling them whom to appoint, and although they might be influenced, by the Acheson committee's analysis for example[45], there was certainly no guarantee that young doctors would be appointed to any vacancies occurring. Furthermore, with the GMSC's rejection of the Acheson proposal that the DHSS should give guidance to the MPC and FPCs on the criteria for selecting candidates to inner city vacancies, even this attempt to influence these bodies was not pursued.

It is, therefore, very likely that one factor in the long delay in responding to the Acheson report was difficulty over the financing of any package of measures, and particularly measures to encourage the retirement of elderly GPs. Here, the DHSS was in a cleft stick, needing some declaration in principle by the GMSC over retirement policy as a lever to overcome Treasury unwillingness to sanction additional expenditure on financial inducements, but in the end making little headway against either the GMSC or the Treasury.

Such an account does at least imply that the DHSS was successful over other aspects of financing primary health care measures in the inner cities. The only proof of this is what was actually announced in October 1983. Here again it is not entirely clear by what stages the £3m one-year plan of November 1982 with unspecified details was converted into a £9m three-year specific plan. It was certainly being rumoured by early 1983 that a £9m three-year plan was being prepared, even that an announcement was to be made in March, and it was claimed that Mr Fowler and Mr Clarke were 'frustrated by the delay'[46]. This was at a time when, as was indicated earlier, Mr Clarke was unable to give the House of Commons any details of the £3m plan for 1983/84.

About this time there was undoubtedly pressure from the medical profession for some more positive response from the government on Acheson and on primary health care in the inner cities generally. The announcement of November 1982 had not been well received. The chairman of the GMSC, Dr John Ball, was reported to have described the £3m then made available as 'the original drop in the ocean'. The Opposition called it 'window dressing'[47], but with increasing rumours that key features of the Acheson proposals, including those dealing with retirement, were unlikely to be carried out, the GMSC took the unusual step of issuing a statement sharply criticising the government for the delay in making a positive response to Acheson. The GMSC, it said, 'accepts no responsibility whatever' for the delay in responding to the Acheson report; it reiterated its position on the main issues raised by the report and ended by saying that 'the GMSC is seriously dismayed at the very extended delay in the response to the Acheson Report'[48]. No doubt part of the object of the statement was to counter the reports that the GMSC had been dragging its heels on the retirement question, for it went out of its way to make explicit that the GMSC was not opposed to inducements to retirement on a voluntary basis. But if part of the object was to stimulate the DHSS or even to strengthen its hand in any discussions with the Treasury, then the statement was a failure. Nearly nine more months passed before the government announced its plans. It is true that a general election intervened, but the same 'ministerial double act' of Fowler and Clarke was dealing with these problems both before and after the election.

There are thus a number of more or less plausible reasons which can be suggested for the delays in the government's response to the Acheson report. They do not seem, however, adequately to explain them. Even after the November 1982 announcement nearly a year elapsed before the full programme of measures was made public. Rumours were rife early in 1983 that, as one headline put it, 'Government to follow Acheson's easy bits'[49]. It is difficult to suppose, therefore, that it was only the practical difficulties, important as these no doubt were, which led to the long delays. It seems evident that primary health care in the inner cities did not have high priority in 1982 and 1983. Just as the publication of the Acheson report had not been enthusiastically welcomed, so the carrying through of a package of measures to support primary health care in the inner cities was not undertaken with any great sense of urgency.

It is perhaps not surprising in the circumstances that the announcement in October 1983 of the £9m package was not greeted with any noticeable enthusiasm. Few went as far as the chairman of the GMSC's practice premises sub-committee, who was reported as saying:

> the Government's response is a very poor show. It's nothing more than a political gesture[50].

There was a general feeling, however, that the response was inadequate[51], 'a small gesture' as the Labour spokesman put it[52]. The bulk of the money was earmarked for three items: higher rate improvement grants for premises; training of health visitors and district nurses; and 'innovative ideas'. Together these accounted for over £7m out of the £9m provided. Other areas which, according to the October 1983 announcement, were likely to benefit included additional incentives to group practice and a scheme for minimum standards for practice premises[53]. Of the major items, that for improvement grants followed Acheson closely except that the higher rate was to be 60 per cent and not 66 per cent as recommended by Acheson; the grants for nurse training were in substitution for the Acheson recommendation of central funding which was rejected. The innovative ideas scheme represented a different approach from that of Acheson. The lesser (in terms of amounts of money) items followed Acheson recommendations, although in modified form. The main question raised by these proposals was clearly how far the money would go and what was likely to be achieved, but three other points raised by the government announcement need to be considered.

The first concerns the areas which were to benefit from the proposals. The criterion adopted was that applying to the government's general inner cities policy, that is, areas which had partnership or programme status, together with the London Docklands Development Corporation, could qualify. This had a slightly distorting effect, particularly in London, where most of the old LCC area qualified except Camden, Kensington and Chelsea, Greenwich and Westminster, but in outer London only Brent and Newham and not, for example, Haringey.

The second point is more important, and concerns the timescale of the proposals. The bulk of the 'Acheson money' was to be spread over the financial years 1983/84 1985/86 and the remainder in 1986/87. No commitment was made beyond that date, but whereas some items, such as the improvement of premises, might reasonably be expected to be carried through in a limited period provided that adequate funds were made available, this was not so obviously true of such items as nurse training or incentives to group practice. Furthermore, there was a problem with central encouragement of innovative ideas in that there was no guarantee that worthwhile innovations would continue to be supported once central support was withdrawn, a fact which the Social Services Committee was later to point out[54]. Altogether, therefore, the government's proposals amounted to a temporary boost to primary health care in the inner cities, but after March 1986 this would once again have to compete for funds through the normal budgetary processes.

The third general point about the government proposals is that a large part of the available funds (roughly one third) was to be allocated not to specific measures, whether directly related to Acheson proposals or not, but to supporting projects put forward by the health authorities. The mechanism was that RHAs were to be asked to consult DHAs and put forward proposals for approval by the DHSS within the total of funds allocated to each RHA for this purpose each year. Although various suggestions were made by the DHSS about the kind of project which might be put forward, the main criterion was that projects should be 'of immediate benefit to primary health care services'. Very often these have been in practice the purchase of items of equipment or the improvement of premises such as clinics or health centres.

Government proposals in detail

The government announcement of October 1983 was not, of course, the last word on the Acheson recommendations. In the final section of this chapter two things will be attempted. First, a brief account will be given of the details of the government's proposals. Secondly, developments since October 1983 which have a bearing on the reception of the Acheson report and, more generally, on problems of primary health care in the inner cities, will be examined. The object is to round off this account of the government's response to the report and to indicate the context within which health authorities have been operating in their attempts to deal with some of the issues raised.

Not surprisingly, details of the various parts of the government's proposals only emerged gradually. Grants for nurse training were the first of the major items, beginning in 1982 with the original £3m allocation. In the first two years (1982/83 and 1983/84) London and the West Midlands did comparatively well out of the allocations, and if this pattern continues something like half the total, or perhaps £5m, will have gone to London.

One reason for the quick start to the nurse training scheme was that it could be put into operation by straightforward administrative action once the idea had been agreed. Measures affecting GPs required formal negotiation of the terms and an official circular to FPCs. The scheme for higher improvements grants was the first to be so treated, a circular being issued in December 1983[55]. The scheme was to run from 1 November 1983 to 31 October 1986, and this immediately gave rise to complaints that insufficient guidance had been provided for the initial five-month period to March 1984 when applications were on a first come, first served basis[56]. A more serious issue was how far the money would go. In 1984/85 each FPC area with a population of 300,000 or more was allocated £33,500; those with populations under 300,000 got £23,000. In 1985/86 the figures were £49,000 and £39,000. A limit of £10,000 grant was set for any individual GP, and £25,000 for any project. As a writer in one of the medical journals pointed out, this and other restrictions which formed part of the scheme would not only tend to discourage all but the most determined GPs but would mean that few would be able to benefit from the grants[57].

As the scheme got under way it emerged that response to it was very varied. Some areas reported little interest whereas others, including City and East London, had more applications than they could meet from their allocations[58]. In addition, there was the general question raised by a scheme of this kind of whether those who had most need of it were the most likely to apply for grants.

As for the 'innovative ideas' scheme, it seems as though the money is being spread even more thinly. In 1983/84 212 projects were approved costing £1.1m or an average of £5,000 a project. Mr Kenneth Clarke referred to:

some excellent innovative schemes . . . some at very low cost.

He also claimed:

no idea is too radical to be considered because we must continue to look for new ways to tackle the problems of the inner city's health services.

In spite of these and other brave words about giving health authorities a chance to try out new ideas and new technology, he admitted that the money could also be used:

to improve the effectiveness and efficiency of existing services[59].

It took rather longer than for either the nurse training or the improvement grant scheme to get agreement on the plan for additional incentives for group practice and on minimum standards for practice premises. The latter is a national scheme but 'Acheson money' is being made available to give a stimulus, particularly for monitoring, in the inner cities. A consequence of the delay in getting agreement on both these schemes is that they will both continue into 1986/87. £600,000 has been allocated for group practice incentives, but no individual doctor can receive more than £4,000 in incentive payments, and the questions which remain to be answered are how far the money will go and whether indeed this kind of incentive is likely to make much impact on the problem. Similarly, a question mark hangs over the minimum standards scheme as to how effective it will prove in practice.

Two additional measures not forming part of the original October 1983 announcement should also be mentioned. Support was to be given to a number of projects devised by the King's Fund, and to certain developments in academic departments of general practice. It is likely that these additional measures owed a good deal to the new Chief Medical Officer at the DHSS from 1 January 1984 who, by a singular irony for the present study, was none other than Professor Donald Acheson. Although nothing had come of the earlier approach by DHSS to the King's Fund on how best to spend £1.2m on improving primary health care in inner London[60], the special concern of the Fund with primary health care in London has been recognised by giving it nearly £4m to undertake three projects on aspects of primary health care identified as important for its future development, such as the employment of development workers for collaboration between FPCs and DHAs.

It will be recalled that the Acheson committee favoured the development of academic departments of general practice, in particular as a means of giving stimulus to general practice in the districts in which the medical schools were situated. Funding of academic posts, however, follows the normal practice under which the University Grants Committee allocates a total sum of money to each university which then decides how the money shall be distributed to the various departments, schools, etc. Within the University of London there was, of course, a powerful medical demand for a share of the available funds, given the large number of teaching hospitals enjoying considerable prestige, but departments of general practice were not generally in a strong position to press for funds against more powerful specialties. The Acheson committee was well aware of this and made a specific recommendation that the UGC should exceptionally indicate to the University of London that funds should be allocated to medical schools specifically for departments of general practice[61]. Remarkably, three posts were in fact created for this purpose in London medical schools in the following years, and this is no doubt connected with the fact that Professor Donald Acheson was chairman of the UGC's medical sub committee in 1982 and 1983. Similarly, the decision to use a small part of the Acheson money to provide a temporary stimulus to the development of relations between departments of general practice and the local community followed his appointment as chief medical officer. Just over £300,000 has been provided for the years 1984/85 1986/87.

Continuing developments in the primary health care field
The £9m has thus been spread over a variety of areas, some directly related to Acheson proposals and some not. But some important Acheson proposals were not mentioned in the October 1983 announcement, particularly those relating to patients' difficulties in getting on to a doctor's list or in making contact once they are on a list[62]. One cannot, however, assume that that is the end of the matter. Certain other developments of the last few years are relevant. In one of the few areas where factual data can be studied, it is possible to trace some changes in general practice, at least in London.

Table 3.1   Percentage of GPs in various age groups, 1975-83

a) under 40	1975	1977	1979	1983
Inner London	18	17	N/A	23
Outer London	21	20	N/A	25
England and Wales	29	30	N/A	36
b) 65 and over	1975	1977	1979	1983
Inner London	18	17	18	14
Outer London	11	12	11	11
England and Wales	6	6	6	5
c) 70 and over	1975	1977	1979	1983
Inner London	10	9	10	8
Outer London	5	6	6	6
England and Wales	3	3	3	2

Sources: Information supplied by the DHSS (1975 and 1983); RCGP, *Survey of Primary Care in London* (1977): Acheson Report, Table 5 (1979).

Table 3.1 shows that there has been some decline in the percentage of elderly doctors in inner London, and a more marked increase of those in younger age groups. From the standpoint of the Acheson committee's analysis the latter figures are particularly encouraging since, although the percentage of GPs under the age of 40 is still very much smaller in inner London than in the country as a whole, there is some suggestion that it may be increasing more rapidly. The trend would need to be studied, however, over several more years.

Table 3.2   Percentage of GPs with small lists

lists	1977 under 1000	1979 under 1000	1983 under 1000
Inner London	7	6	5
Outer London	3	3	3
England & Wales	2	1	2

Sources: as for Table 3.1: Acheson Report, Table 9.

Again, one might describe these figures as mildly encouraging from the Acheson committee's point of view, particularly in that they show a marked decline in the proportion of doctors with very small lists.

Table 3.3   Percentage of GPs not in group practice

	1977	1979	1983
Inner London	61	59	54
Outer London	50	48	41
England and Wales	30	28	24

Sources: RCGP, *Survey*: Acheson Report, Table 3: DHSS.

Here, although the trend in inner London is towards group practice, it is not as marked as in the country generally and a majority of GPs are not in group practice, compared with only about a quarter in the country generally.

It is not suggested that one can draw any very pronounced conclusions from these figures, still less that so far as they show tendencies in the direction desired by the Acheson committee those tendencies are attributable to the effects of the committee's report. They are presented here merely to show that in the post-Acheson period there are more younger doctors and fewer elderly ones than when the committee started work, fewer doctors with small lists and more working in group practices.

There have been some developments on particular Acheson proposals, most notably on the vexed question of retirement for GPs. As has been seen earlier, it is not quite true to say that retirement of GPs was an unmentionable subject before Acheson reported. It is true, however, that a fixed age of retirement, such as applied, for example, to hospital doctors, was regarded as out of the question so far as the spokesmen of the medical profession were concerned. What the profession wanted, as the report of the New Charter Working Group acknowledged, was to continue the freedom for the individual GP to retire when he chose but to make it possible for him not to have to go on working for financial reasons[63]. This was a kind of halfway house position, as the GMSC made clear in its response to the report of the Royal Commission on the National Health Service, in which the profession was prepared to consider an assisted voluntary retirement scheme for GPs with small lists aged over 65, but was not prepared to discuss the feasibility of a compulsory retiring age[64].

This position was re-affirmed in the discussions with the DHSS following the report of the Acheson committee, but some shift of view among members of the profession has since become apparent. In 1984 the conference of Local Medical Committees for the first time asked the GMSC to investigate a normal age of retirement for GPs[65].

This was followed up at the BMA's annual conference, although it was clear that there were still considerable differences of view, some GPs arguing that there should be no compulsion to retire whereas others thought that it was wrong for GPs to carry on working after the age of 65[66]. It will be interesting to see what emerges from the GMSC on this question, although it is unlikely that it will want to say anything very positive until after the appearance of the government's Green Paper, discussed below. Again, the difficult question is how far the Acheson proposals acted as a stimulus to this shift in view within the profession so that it is at least now willing to discuss retirement policy. Other factors are certainly present. One of the 1984 motions, for example, favoured encouragement for GPs to retire at 65 'in view of the increasing unemployment of medical graduates'. The employment situation has indeed figured prominently in recent medical discussions. Again, at the 1984 LMC conference, for example, rising medical unemployment was used as an argument for pressing urgently to achieve the BMA's long standing target of an average list size of 1700 patients[67].

One of the more important developments in primary health care generally has been the changed status of family practitioner committees. Since 1 April 1985 FPCs have become independent authorities within the National Health Service directly accountable to the DHSS. Much of the controversy which surrounded the introduction of this change centred on the question of whether it would help or hinder better planning of primary health care at local level. Many favoured integration with DHAs for this purpose. Now that the change has been made, two major questions arise: whether the relationship between FPCs and DHAs can lead to an effective partnership (or collaboration as the DHSS seems to prefer to call it) in the planning and provision of services; and whether the present government's concern with value for money can stimulate greater management efficiency in the FPC sector. It seems likely that one outcome will be more central control particularly in financial matters, but it is difficult to predict at this stage what the longer-term consequences will be.

Although the measures announced in October 1983 flowing from the Acheson committee's report are still continuing, the main focus of interest so far as government policy on primary health care is concerned has now shifted to a proposed Green Paper[68]. First reports suggested that this was to be very wide-ranging, taking in assessments of the future work load of GPs, the scope for expansion of community nursing, methods of controlling the costs of the family practitioner services and so on. Particularly interesting in the present context is the fact that retirement policy was said to be one of the matters to be considered. Indeed an unnamed DHSS source was quoted as saying:

> this is an area which has to be looked at. The whole purpose of the Green Paper is to consult, not to dictate. But retirement policy must be on the agenda[69].

Originally announced for the summer of 1984, and promised by the Secretary of State for the autumn of that year[70], the Green Paper has become something of a mirage and has still (June 1986) not appeared. If and when it does eventually appear it may be still wider in scope and include proposals on retirement of GPs at 65 or 70 specifically to improve primary care in inner cities[71]. It would be pointless to speculate on why the Green Paper has taken so long to appear, even though a writer in the *British Medical Journal* has rather cynically remarked that a year behind schedule is about normal and more than a year 'good going even for the Department of Health and Social Security'[72]. The arrival of a new chief medical officer with a close interest in primary health care, especially in the inner cities, Mr Fowler's preoccupation with the series of social security reviews[73], Ministers' embroilment with the GMSC and the pharmaceutical industry over the proposal to limit the list of drugs to be prescribed by GPs—all these may well at various times have played a part in delaying the appearance of the Green Paper.

What is important in the present context is that, so far as the future of primary health care in the inner cities is concerned, the Green Paper has become the main focus of interest for the future of government policy. Within the next year the last of the Acheson money will have been spent, with whatever temporary or permanent consequences for primary health care in the inner cities this may bring something still to be assessed in the future. But beyond that, both in time and scale of development, it will be the outcome of whatever proposals the Green Paper contains which will largely determine whether there will be an effective policy response from the government to the continuing problems of primary health care in the inner cities.

This is not to say, of course, that the Green Paper is everything and that one can ignore what is happening elsewhere. The GMSC, as has been indicated earlier, had, even when the Acheson committee was still in operation, initiated, through its working group on under-privileged areas, a new approach to the identification of such areas which could have considerable consequences for the way in which GPs working in inner city areas, among others, are paid. Following the report of the Acheson inquiry, the working group was reconstituted as a sub-committee of the GMSC and has done a great deal of work on the practical problems of identifying and testing the validity of the criteria needed. A formula has been devised for identifying in quantifiable terms under-privileged areas whether in inner cities or elsewhere, for example, some of the industrial areas of South Wales. This approach has received general endorsement at the annual medical conference and by the GMSC. The next stage is to see what the relationship is between such deprivation and, for example, the level of resources allocated to primary health care[74].

In spite of the considerable progress which this initiative has made, its translation into practical consequences still lies some way in the future. The implementation of the Black report on inequalities in health seems an even remoter possibility. Nevertheless, the report is not dead, as a subject of debate at least, even after five years, and some members of the BMA think that the association should be campaigning for its implementation even after its brusque rejection by the government in 1980[75]. Again, if the Black report were to be taken up it would obviously have profound consequences for primary health care in the inner cities.

One other possibility ought also to be mentioned here. The Green Paper, it is suggested in some quarters, will be 'radical'[76]. But how radical? To some people it has always seemed that the problems of primary health care in the inner cities require a move away from the consensus approach which has hitherto characterised much discussion of the issue and most of the actual measures which have been tried. In particular, the idea of a salaried service for GPs in place of the present independent contractor status has seemed to some a necessary move in any attempts to improve primary health care in the inner cities. That idea has, of course, never been endorsed by the medical profession, although the BMA did go so far as to suggest in 1965 that it might be one option for GPs; even this was subsequently withdrawn[77]. If a salaried service were, however, to be proposed by the DHSS as a replacement of the existing system there is no doubt that it would be strenuously resisted by the profession.

It would hardly be worth mentioning the possibility but for two reasons. The first is that it was rumoured that the chief medical Officer, Professor Donald Acheson, was at least sympathetic to the idea of a salaried service. Indeed, the former Minister of State at the Department, Sir Gerard Vaughan, in an article in 1984 shortly after Professor Acheson took over, seemed to be trying to warn him off the idea. After saying that it was 'widely believed' that Professor Acheson favoured a state salaried service, he went on:

I don't believe this is so. I believe he has seen far too much of the benefit from the present system to want to disturb it[78].

However, whatever the origin of Sir Gerard's view, there is no evidence that Professor Acheson wishes to move in the direction of a salaried service.

The second reason is a rather more general one. A recent writer in the *British Medical Journal* has noted that three times recently the government has seemed to be moving away from the traditional consensus approach, or, as he put it:

has used its political muscle to bounce major changes on the profession and the NHS[79]. One might deduce from this that the possibility of a salaried service is not so remote as it generally appears. On the other hand, it should be noted that the three instances referred to (the Griffiths management reforms, the attempt to strengthen control over the use of deputising services, restrictions on prescribing) are all very close to the present government's preoccupation with economy and efficiency. It is by no means certain that a move to a salaried service would be either cheaper or more efficient, although it would certainly make it easier to control the at present notoriously uncontrollable expenditure on family practitioner services[80], and bring nearer the Treasury's evident aim to impose cash limits on them[81]. Nor, of course, whatever Professor Acheson's views may be, is it a foregone conclusion that he will be able to convince colleagues and Ministers to support them.

All this is to suggest only that we have passed out of a strictly Acheson phase, the phase when the main question was what response the government would make to the Acheson report, and into a different phase when the future of primary health care in general must be the prime focus and the particular problems of inner cities have to be viewed in that light. Perhaps it would be better to say that the Acheson phase has merged into this wider phase, and certainly one cannot simply dismiss Acheson ideas because they did not find a place in the October 1983 proposals; retirement policy is an obvious example.

There remains, nevertheless, the question of assessing the impact of the Acheson report so far as it is possible to do so at this stage. To do that realistically requires more than an examination of major policy issues. The following chapter, therefore, considers what has been happening in the regions, districts and family practioner committees of inner London, and how far the Acheson report has influenced decisions there.

References

1   cf. HC Deb. 29 July 1982, vol. 28, col.1369.
2   *Acute Hospital Services in London*, London Advisory Group, January 1981, paras 14, 15. The chairman (Sir John Habbakuk) in his covering letter also stressed the view that 'a large proportion' of savings in the acute field should go to other services.
3   *The Development of Health Services in London*, London Advisory Group, May 1981, paras, 3,5,14.
4   See Chapter 2, p.23.
5   Dr (now Sir) Gerard Vaughan, HC Deb. 18 May 1981, vol.5, WA41.
6   Rudolf Klein, *The Politics of the National Health Service*, Longman, 1983, p.128.
7   Mr Tony Newton speaking in a debate on health care in inner London, HC Deb. 29 July 1982, vol. 28, col.1369.
8   *Acute Hospital Services in London*, LHPC, 1979, Table G3: *Towards a Balance*, LHPC, 1980, paras 18-20 and Table T2.
9   Whether and to what extent there has been real growth in NHS expenditure in recent years has become a matter of some dispute. Much turns on whether one regards the demographic and other factors which make increased expenditure necessary simply in order to maintain existing standards of services as 'real' growth or merely maintenance of the service. See *The Lancet*, 19 March 1983, pp.659-60: HC Deb., 25 March 1983, vol. 39, col. 1242 (Mr K. Clarke): Social Services Committee, Fourth Report, 1983/84 (HC 395), Table 1 and para. 13: HC Deb. 14 May 1985, vol. 79, WA 1189: Klim McPherson, 'The political argument on health costs', *BMJ*, 8 June 1985, pp.1679-80.
10 *Acute Hospital Services in London*, LAG, 1981, Foreword, para 5.
11 G.H. Ward and P.A. West, 'What price the London Hospital Plan', *BMJ*, 14 March 1981, pp.922-3.
12 Without going into the complexities of the arrangements for remunerating general practitioners, the essential point is that the Review Body determines a figure of average net pay and prices the various fees and allowances to achieve this. If additional payments to London (or inner city) doctors were to be taken into account for average pay purposes, this would be at the expense of those not qualifying for such payments. This is why the BMA favours the exclusion

of payments not open to all doctors in the calculation of average net pay. (See *Report of New Charter Working Group*, BMA, February 1979, para. 7.2.)

13 See, for example, *BMJ*, 1 June 1974, p.83: 29 June 1974, p.141: 31 July 1976, p.33: 6 August 1977, p.404: 15 July 1978, p.225.

14 *The Lancet*, 19/26 December 1981, p.1431.

15 i.e. 500 x one third (the extra cost of 66 and two thirds per cent as against 33 and a third per cent grants) x £30,000.

16 i.e. 400 x £18,000.

17 *The Lancet, op.cit.*

18 *Report of the Working Group on Inequalities in Health*, DHSS, 1980.

19 See statement by Mr Heseltine, HC Deb. 9 February 1981, vol. 998, cols 603-4.

20 *BMJ*, 7 February 1981, pp.489-90.

21 See *Pulse*, 13 February 1982, p.1.

22 'Primary care in inner London: inadequate and exposed', *BMJ*, 30 May 1981, pp.1739-40.

23 Rodney Deitch in *The Lancet*, 30 May 1981, pp.1219-20.

24 See *Pulse*, for example, 30 May 1981, pp.4-5.

25 It is also significant that in October 1982 the GMSC and the RCGP addressed a joint letter to the Secretary of State urging an early response to the Acheson report.

26 See Report, Annex 8: no fewer than 40 per cent of the elderly GPs who answered the questionnaire gave their desire to continue working as their sole reason for not retiring, and a further 35 per cent gave that together with inability to afford to retire.

27 Although answering arrangements did not figure in the government's eventual response to Acheson, the GMSC later drew up a code of practice and guidance for GPs, *BMJ*, 1 December 1984, p.1555.

28 See *BMJ*, 5 February 1983, p.493.

29 cf. *Doctor*, 23 June 1983, p.9.

30 *Times Health Supplement*, 18 December 1981, p.1. cf. *The Lancet*, 19/26 December 1981, p.1430.

31 Mr Norman Fowler, HC Deb. 8 November 1982, vol. 31, cols 329-31.

32 HC Deb. 6 December 1982, vol. 33, cols 603-4.

33 HC Deb. 16 February 1983, vol. 37, WA 197: 9 March 1983, vol. 38, WA 419; 15 March 1983, vol. 39, WA 141: Standing Committee B, 28 April 1983, col. 817.

34 Mr Tony Newton, Under Secretary of State, DHSS, HC Deb. 29 July 1982, vol. 28, cols 1369-70.

35 Nearly £1m of this first 'Acheson money' was, however, made available for nurse training, some of it in 1982/83.

36 Rodney Deitch, 'General Practice in Inner Cities', *The Lancet*, 5 February 1983, p.308.

37 Rodney Deitch, *The Lancet*, 23 July 1983, p.232.

38 *General Practitioner*, 12 November 1982, p.1.

39 *Pulse*, 20 November 1982, p.7: *Guardian*, 4 May 1983 ('Treasury blocks GP cash'): *Doctor*, 23 June 1983, p.9: *The Lancet*, 14 April 1984, p.862.

40 House of Commons, Social Services Committee, Fourth Report, Session 1983/84, (HC 395), para. 9.

41 The Binder Hamlyn report has not so far been published, although it was completed over two years ago.

42 HC 395, 1983/84, question 41.

43 Report, Annex 8.

44 HC Standing Committee B, Health and Social Services and Social Security Adjudications Bill, 20th sitting, 28 April 1983, cols 816-7; he was speaking on a clause moved by the Opposition which would have had the effect of incorporating many of the Acheson proposals into the Bill.

45 MPC did, in fact, modify its guidance to FPCs to make it easier for young doctors to be considered for vacancies. (See previous reference, col. 816).

46 See *The Lancet*, 5 February 1983, p.308: *General Practitioner*, 11 March 1983, p.1.

47 *Doctor*, 27 January 1983, p.1: Standing Committee B, 28 April 1983, col. 813.

48 See report in *BMJ*, 5 February 1983, p.493.

49 *The Health Services*, 11 March 1983, p.1.

50 Dr Arnold Elliott in *Doctor*, 17 November 1983, p.2.

51 'Grossly inadequate' in the view of Dr John Ball, chairman of the GMSC, *BMJ*, 10 December 1983, p.1818.

52 Mrs Gwyneth Dunwoody, HC Deb. 27 October 1983, vol. 47, col. 507.

53 The final break down of the £9m is likely to be:

Health authority projects   £3.3m
(innovative ideas)

Higher rate improvement grants	£2.4m
Training extra health visitors and district nurses	£1.5m
Incentives to group practice	£0.6m
King's Fund projects	£0.5m
Minimum standards, premises	£0.4m
Academic departments	£0.3m

54 HC 395, para. 35.

55 HN (83)36.

56 See the comments by Dr John Ball, chairman of the GMSC, in *BMJ*, 10 December 1983, p.1818.

57 Olivia Timbs, 'Hurry for inner city cash', *Medeconomics*, January; 1984, p.25.

58 Jacky Law, 'Slow GPs miss city cash', *Medeconomics*, September 1984, p.34.

59 HC Deb. 25 June 1984, vol. 62, WA 359-60. It seems that the money was allocated in 1983/84 to RHAs according to the populations of their partnership and programme authorities: the Thames regions on this basis received approximately 20 per cent of the total allocation of £1.2m.

60 The King's Fund suggested that a trust fund should be set up to decide how the money should be spent but this ingenious idea ran into difficulties over questions of accountability, and was not pursued further.

61 Acheson Report, paras 10, 14, 16. For UGC policy on specific allocations see House of Commons, Expenditure Committee, Second Report, Session 1970/71 (HC 545), pp.194-8, para 8: and Education, Science and Arts Committee, Fifth Report Session 1979/80 (HC 787), pp.43-4.

62 For other reasons the government in 1983 and 1984 pursued a policy of tighter controls over GP deputising services, the manner of which provoked a well publicised confrontation with the GMSC.

63 *Report of the New Charter Working Group, op.cit.*, para 7.12.

64 *BMJ*, 6 October 1979, pp.878-9.

65 *BMJ*, 7 July 1984, p.64.

66 *BMJ*, 21 July 1984, p.202. In 1985 the LMC conference reaffirmed its opposition to a compulsory retirement age, *BMJ*, 29 June 1985, p.1978.

67 *BMJ*, 2 July 1983, p.70.

68 HC Deb. 6 April 1984, vol.57, WA 689-91.

69 Rodney Deitch, 'Another Scrutiny for Primary Care', *The Lancet*, 14 April 1984, pp.862-3; cf. *The Times*, 4 April 1984, p.1.

70 HC 395, question 4107.

71 Nicholas Timmins, 'GPs may be able to advertise', *The Times*, 8 April 1985.

72 William Russell, 'BMA and DHSS back on an even keel?' *BMJ*, 13 April 1985, p.1156; and 'That evermore elusive Green Paper', *BMJ*, 22 June 1985.

73 cf. William Russell, 'Green Paper on general practice delayed until 1985', *BMJ*, 3 November 1984, p.1237: he suggests that even Mr Clarke was taken by surprise at the decision to postpone the Green Paper.

74 See GMSC Reports: 1982, paras.77-8; 1983, paras.75-7; 1984, paras.96-8; 1985, paras.178-81.

75 The view of the Junior Members' Forum, as reported in *BMJ*, 13 April 1985, p.1157.

76 William Russell in *BMJ*, 13 April 1985, p.1156.

77 'A Charter for the Family Doctor Service', *BMJ Supp.*, 13 March 1965, para. 4 (vii): *Report of New Charter Working Group, op.cit.*, paras 6.9-12.

78 'Why GPs should worry', *Pulse*, 18 February 1984, p.29.

79 'Scrutator', 'The Week', *BMJ* 13 April 1985, p.1155.

80 cf. HC 395, para. 11.

81 It is rumoured that the Binder Hamlyn report does not offer much comfort to the Treasury on this but it is still not clear whether the report will be published at the same time as the Green Paper.

CHAPTER 4 THE ACHESON REPORT AS A CATALYST TO ACTION

Introduction

In the last chapter we discussed the government's response to the Acheson report and described the context within which health authorities, family practitioner committees, and others concerned with primary health care have been operating in their attempts to deal with some of the issues in this field. The report provided some stimulus to change, and a limited amount of additional money from central government. However, the significance of all the recommendations contained in the report does not lie in the response of the DHSS alone. The implementation of some proposals is dependent upon the attitudes, reactions and initiatives of health authorities, family practitioner committees, local authorities and others concerned with the provision of primary health care.

One of the aspirations of the Acheson report was 'to create conditions in which local initiatives can flourish and the flexible and thoughtful application of our proposals will lead to real improvements in services to patients'[1]. This chapter examines how far the report has encouraged such conditions, thereby providing a text for, or a catalyst to, the process of change in areas not directly dependent upon DHSS decisions. It also examines what has been achieved with the limited amount of money, and what changes and improvements have taken place in five inner London districts and in the three regions within which they fall. The responses of the FPCs to the criticisms levelled at them in the Acheson report are also considered. This chapter does not evaluate the changes which have taken place but merely describes some of the developments and assesses the impact of the report at local level.

A report prepared by a working group of the Royal College of General Practitioners has shown that certain social and medical characteristics tend to occur together in inner London, but the most demonstrable and striking difference is between the East End and West End London boroughs[2]. In the East End boroughs there is a relatively stable but very deprived population living in conditions of environmental decay. There are higher proportions of social classes III, IV and V, more economically active males who are sick, higher infant mortality rates and more deaths from lung cancer. In West End boroughs (Kensington and Chelsea, Westminster, Camden and Hammersmith) the population is generally less stable, with lower proportions of married couple households, higher proportions of one-person households and bed-sitters, high population density, a highly mobile population (including tourists and visitors), a high crime rate, and high suicide and mental illness admission rates. There are, of course, close links between ill-health and, on the one hand, high mortality and social deprivation, on the other, as was shown by the Black report[3].

Bearing these factors in mind we looked at three 'East End' health districts (City and Hackney, Tower Hamlets and Camberwell) and two 'West End' health districts (Bloomsbury and Victoria—from 1 April 1985 part of Riverside Health Authority) to see how the Acheson proposals have been adopted and interpreted in the light of local circumstances. We begin, however, by examining developments in the three regional health authorities, which cover the five districts, namely, North East, North West and South East Thames RHAs, in order to see what impact the Acheson report had on the development of strategic plans and initiatives within these regions.

Impact of Acheson at the regional level

Regional strategies for primary health care reflect national policies. These stress the priority to be given to care in the community and shifting the balance from hospital to community care; the need to strengthen primary care and community health services; the importance of primary health care teams; and the need for better collaboration and co-ordination between health services, family practitioner committees, local authorities and the voluntary sector. But, despite common themes, the approaches adopted by the regions vary, as do their emphases. These are obviously shaped by local circumstances, priorities and the individuals involved.

Many of the ideas in the Acheson report were not new and others had advocated similar ideas before. *The NE Thames RHA*, for example, which covers City and Hackney, Tower Hamlets and Bloomsbury districts, has, over the past nine years, given particular attention to improving primary health care, especially in the 'East End' of London. In 1976 a regional working party on primary health care commissioned various studies on general practice and community nursing services[4]. The working party's recommendations were reflected in the Regional Strategic Plan (1977/8) in a programme of short- and longer-term measures to remedy deficiencies in primary care. Two important and innovative elements of this programme were the establishment of a Centre for the Study of Primary Care[5] in the East End which opened in 1983; and the establishment of a post of general practice facilitator. The Centre was conceived as a focus for teaching and research in the field of primary care but especially in the area of teamwork within primary care. It was envisaged that the presence of the Centre would act as a stimulus to local primary care and promote improvements in the quality of care, including the recruitment of better qualified and motivated staff.

The post of general practice facilitator was established on an experimental basis in order to determine the value of employing an experienced GP, well versed in ways and means of improving general practice premises and organisation, to assist GPs to improve, where necessary, their standards of practice. The post was funded by the Hackney/Islington Inner City Partnership for a two-year period and Dr Arnold Elliott, who had been party to the invention of the concept, was appointed to the post. This initiative was subsequently welcomed by the Acheson committee which recommended that the four Thames RHAs jointly set up and finance a team of co-ordinators for inner London.

So the thinking which the NE Thames Region had done in this field had a significant impact on the Acheson committee, and the region's analysis of the problems and their prescriptions for action were very similar to those which were later contained in the Acheson report. However, the regions, and particularly the NE Thames RHA, had hoped for a more positive response from the government and greater resources than were forthcoming. Continuing themes in its 1984/93 Strategic Plan are improvements in community nursing numbers and attachments and in the long-term attachments to general practices on a 'patchwork' basis; improvement of links between primary and hospital care; provision of diagnostic facilities for GPs; creation of joint administrative appointments with matching family practitioner committees in order to promote integrated management and planning; a further consideration of the general practitioner facilitator role as another means of promoting links between community health service and general practice; and encouragement of family practitioner committees to improve general practice services. For this region, therefore, the Acheson report backed the ideas which were already in currency and provided further impetus for change.

The *SE Thames RHA* set up a members' panel on primary health care in April 1983 to study primary care in the South East and to recommend measures to the region to assist its development within the funds and manpower likely to be made available, and with special reference to the problems of inner London in the light of the Acheson and Harding reports; to identify priorities for action in the next three years and ten years; and to formulate policies to encourage other agencies within the region to meet agreed priorities[6]. Such a comprehensive and full review had not been attempted by the SE Thames region before. The panel concentrated on the special needs of general practitioners, training and continuing education, community nursing in inner London, accident and emergency departments and information. The recommendations of the panel were accepted by the region early in 1984 and incorporated in the Regional Strategy for 1985-94. The strategy document stated:

> The four areas [needs of GPs; training and continuing education; community nursing in inner London; accident and emergency departments] described above arise out of a preliminary study of the Acheson Report's recommendations on Primary Health Care in Inner London. They are not comprehensive. They are not quantified. But they provide a general direction which Districts are asked to follow, whilst both the members' panel

and District Health Authorities work to collate wider information on deficiencies and development needs across the whole range of primary health care services and to consider how health authorities can work with other agencies to implement change[7].

In the SE Thames region it would appear that the Acheson and Harding reports provided an impetus for consideration of primary care issues and pointed the region towards a more strategic look at primary care.

The *NW Thames RHA* published a regional strategy in September 1984 for consultation[8]. The document defined in broad terms the main issues in primary care in the region and identified strategic issues for further discussion. The underlying themes were similar to those which appeared in the strategic documents of other regions. *A propos* the Acheson report the document stated that 'In general the RHA should work more closely with District Health Authorities and Family Practitioner Committees to define priorities and policies in primary health care'[9]. One of the main developments in this region is the funding of a GP facilitator, but unlike the NE Thames Region's experiment where the emphasis was on GP premises, the emphasis of this appointment— which has been delayed due to reorganisation of FPCs—will be on practice organisation, management, post-graduate teaching and research.

On the question of allocation of Acheson money, the following categories were suggested to the regions by the DHSS:

> Examples might include projects to improve the primary health provision projects to provide additional training for staff working in the community and primary health care field, including pyschiatric nurses, development of evening and night nursing services, improvements to the supply of nursing aids and equipments, local research projects or pilot studies aimed at improving the effectiveness of primary health care services either generally or for specific client groups or improving liaison and co-operation with other services[9].

In practice the regions adopted varied criteria for allocating the Acheson money. The NW Thames region allocated money to projects concerned with health education and health information. This region took particular care to ensure that the Acheson money went to those projects which would improve the *quality of primary health care*. For example, the specialist in community medicine personally interviewed all the applicants and gave priority to those projects where the applicants had consulted others involved in primary care and which would improve links between hospitals and the community. The NE Thames Region spent the money on projects concerned with *general medical services* but it is not clear what criteria were used for allocating the money. The SE Thames Region made a large investment in microcomputers and related projects to improve *primary care information systems*. This region also allocated money to those projects which it assessed would directly benefit primary care.

This brief examination of the three regions illustrates that the Acheson report was considered by the three regions, and, to varying degrees, influenced their thinking and gave backing to the ideas and trends which were already in currency. We now turn to examine the responses of each of the five districts included in our study.

The impact of Acheson at district level
The characteristics of five DHAs

Before looking at the impact of the Acheson recommendations at district level we shall briefly describe the social needs in the five inner London districts which were the subject of this study. Comparative statistics for the five districts are shown in Table 4.1, but their principal characteristics can be summarised as follows.

City and Hackney is a highly deprived district. The prevalence of factors such as high unemployment levels, significantly higher proportion of social classes IV and V, and poor housing conditions all have an effect on the health status of the population. There is a high infant mortality rate, and a high incidence of illness among the economically active. Social deprivation also increases the levels of mortality and morbidity and generates extra demands on community and primary health care services. The district also has a mobile population, including the homeless and rootless who may be unable or unwilling to register with a GP. Many of the GPs are elderly. They have small lists, often operate single-handed in lock-up and otherwise inadequate premises. This leads to some patients experiencing difficulty in obtaining a GP, leading to their making greater use of accident and emergency services than is the case elsewhere.

Like City and Hackney district, *Tower Hamlets Health District* has extremely poor social, economic and environmental conditions. The district has very high unemployment and a large number of single-parent families. Unlike other inner London districts, the population in Tower Hamlets is expected to increase from just below 150,000 to nearly 160,000 by 1991. The number of elderly is expected to increase marginally. The district also has a large ethnic minority (mainly Bengali) population. The general level of health in Tower Hamlets is poor. Standardised mortality rates are high and the infant and perinatal mortality rates and the high proportion of low birth weight babies are a cause for concern.

Camberwell District Health Authority suffers from all the features of inner city deprivation. Most parts of the district suffer from high levels of overcrowding, poor housing conditions, large numbers of single-parent families, high population mobility, unemployment and mental illness. However, the pattern in the district is by no means uniform; some areas like Dulwich are relatively prosperous. In other parts of the district, poverty and social inequality have worsened as the economic recession has deepened. Poor social and economic conditions encourage illnesses like chest infections, asthma and mental illness. Camberwell also has a high proportion of ethnic minorities with special diseases, for example, sickle cell anaemia and thalassaemia. Deprivation generates disproportionate demands on primary health services and some-

Table 4.1 Characteristics of five district health authorities

	Elderly		Children		Economic		Housing		Migration	
	Living alone	Over 65	Under 5	One parent families	Un-skilled	Unem-ployed	House-hold with lack of amen-ities	Over-crowded	Change in add-ress	Ethnic minor-ities
City & Hackney	6	14	7	5	7	15	9	18	11	27
Tower Hamlets	6	14	7	4	11	16	6	22	12	20
Camberwell	6	14	6	5	8	13	6	13	12	22
Bloomsbury	10	20	4	3	6	10	7	12	17	11
Victoria	9	16	4	2	4	9	8	11	22	7

Source: P. Rice, D. Irving and D. Davies, *Information about District Health Authorities in England from 1981 Census*, King's Fund Publication, 1984.

Notes:
Elderly. Living alone: Pensioners (females over 60, males over 65) living alone as a percentage of all residents in private households. Over 65: People aged 65 or more as a percentage of all residents in private households. *Children.* Under 5: Children under 5 as a percentage of all residents in private households. One-Parent Families: People in households consisting of one person over 16 and one or more children under 16 as a percentage of all residents in private households. *Economic.* Unskilled: People in households headed by a person in socio-economic group II as a percentage of all residents in private households. Unemployed: People aged 16 or more seeking work or temporarily sick as a percentage of the total economically active population. *Housing.* Households with lack of amenities: People in households lacking exclusive use of a bath and inside W.C. as a percentage of all residents in private households. Overcrowded: People in households living at more than one person per room as a percentage of all residents in private households. *Migration.* Changed Address: People aged 1 or over with a usual address one year before the census different from present usual address as a percentage of total residents. Ethnic minorities: People in households headed by a person born in the New Commonwealth or Pakistan as a percentage of all residents in private households.

times leads to heavy use of accident and emergency services. Two informants stated that the riots of 1981 underlined the social situation in Camberwell and that the Scarman report[10] had as much impact as the Acheson report, if not more. The riots generated a feeling that 'something must be done'.

Within the *Bloomsbury District Health Authority* there are diverse neighbourhoods of widely varying socio-economic groups with different health needs. The northern part of the district is predominantly residential and the southern part has a high concentration of offices, hotels, restaurants and shops. There are several underground stations and British Rail termini, which bring a large number of commuters into the district each day. The presence of colleges of the University of London and other educational establishments increases the student population in Bloomsbury. The population density within the district varies considerably. In some pockets, social deprivation and concentration of ethnic minorities are marked. The district has a disproportionately high elderly population and low child population. The diverse characteristics are reflected in the very different residential arrangements; in some wards there is a heavy concentration of council accommodation and in others high owner occupation. The level of infant and perinatal mortality, however, is low. Bloomsbury, therefore, has many of the features which create high demands upon GP services, and it has a high proportion of doctors working in single-handed practices. The high property costs in Central London make it especially difficult for GPs to provide services from well-appointed, attractive accommodation with adequate space for a group practice to operate or for other health professionals to be closely associated with GPs. This leads to a major problem in creating an accessible service.

The population in *Victoria (now part of Riverside) District* is highly mobile. Migration into the area tends to be of young single people, and there is a relative under-representation of married persons, who migrate out of the area. This in turn results in a very low number of children in the district. The proportion of elderly people is about equal to the national average, but the outward migration of young married couples increases the social isolation of old people. The overall mortality amongst residents is not significantly high but a high incidence of suicide has been a feature of the district for some years. It also has a large number of commuters coming to work in Westminster as well as tourists and visitors. In the face of these characteristics Victoria has all the problems associated with inner city general practice highlighted by the Acheson report. In addition, the high mobility of population results in a high rate of turnover of general practitioner lists and a number of claims for temporary residents.

Improving GP services

Because of acute problems in the East End (prior to Acheson) the Primary Health Care (Hackney) sub-Group was established in 1978 by the Officers Steering Group of the Partnership under the chairmanship of Dr M. Salkind, a local GP and chairman of the District Planning Team (Primary Care), now Professor of General Practice at St Bartholomew's Hospital. The report of this sub-group[11] had recommended a retirement policy for GPs, and urged the

74

Medical Practices Committee to allow a GP in a group practice who was considering retirement to take on a replacement partner for up to eighteen months before his retirement on the understanding that the practice would revert to its original number of partners on the date set for the retirement of the GP in question. It also recommended the MPC to adopt a more positive approach to applications for an additional partner where practice size had increased; usually by the time single-handed GPs retire, their practices are so small that the list is dispersed among surrounding GPs rather than advertised. The sub-group's report also pointed out that some surgery premises in Hackney failed to reach the standard of the DHSS guidance on practice accommodation and were too small to allow for attachments of community nursing staff. On the question of premises, the sub-group recommended that a survey be made of the state of GP premises and that the FPC should take a more positive role in approaching GPs about grants and loans available for improvements to premises; that a firm of architects be retained to give specialised assistance to GPs considering extending their premises and in particular to give advice on the feasibility of a reconstruction scheme and funding arrangements; that the powers of the General Practice Finance Corporation be extended to allow the corporation to buy suitable practice premises and lease them to GPs; and that informal machinery should be set up to provide a forum in which to discuss individual problems as they arise. Other recommendations included greater development of health centres, better organisation of GP practices with better patients' records and use of computers, inservice training for receptionists, and establishment of a daily service to collect samples from GP surgeries and clinic premises and deliver them to pathology laboratories. The report also recommended a package of incentives to encourage recruitment of community nursing staff and easing of some of the obstacles, like the large number of single-handed GPs and the inadequate nature of GP premises, in order to facilitate community nurse attachments to GPs and further develop the primary health care team concept.

The Acheson report echoed these recommendations. In any event, some of the proposals contained in the Acheson report were already being implemented in the City and Hackney Health District. For example, there was already university involvement in primary care. Three lecturers in General Practice were attached to the Department of General Practice at St Bartholomew's Hospital. These were funded by Partnership money, initially for three years, and had a direct relationship to the early work of the sub-group.

Against such a background, what impact did Acheson have? Let us take general practice and related services first. At a concrete level the Acheson money enabled the Department of General Practice at St Bartholomew's to appoint an additional senior lecturer, lecturer and secretary, thus increasing the number of students who could be taught. It also enabled the department to develop a research programme and increase liaison with the community. Issues which the department has been looking at include use of computers by general practices, provision for the homeless and rootless and family therapy.

At another level Acheson provided a context for developments to improve and develop both the services provided by GPs and facilities for them. For instance, the City and Hackney DHA demonstrated the priority it attached to primary health care by employing a Primary Care Liaison Officer in 1983. This appointment was a direct result of Acheson. The officer was based in the Community Unit, and the post was funded through a grant to the district from Inner City Partnership funds. The responsibilities of the post were to assess problems facing providers and users of services, to establish links with primary care staff and improve liaison and to contribute to district strategy through participation in its Primary Care Strategy Group. The Primary Care Liaison Officer encouraged GPs to participate in monthly lunchtime seminars. Related to this policy of integration through discussion and information sharing was the production of a District 'Primary Health Care Bulletin', which is the main vehicle in which forthcoming meetings in the district are publicised; in the past this had been done on an individual, unco-ordinated basis. It is claimed that having been provided with opportunities to meet, GPs have become interested in planning issues.

Other work of the Liaison Officer included planning an extended pathology laboratory courier service for GPs practising elsewhere than in health centres (the courier service is presently operating throughout the district, but the expansion of the service depends on Inner City Partnership Funds), looking at health centre catchment areas, and preparing a guide to the services provided by local GPs, together with a location map for distribution to libraries and social services departments. To improve access to services the district purchased two mobile caravans, one for clinical services and the other for health education activities.

The Tower Hamlets DHA, on the other hand, obtained funds from the King's Fund for a three-year Primary Care Development Project (1983-86) to help resolve practical problems in the delivery of effective primary care and to support new initiatives. The project initially concentrated on three main areas: looking at the practical problems of GPs; encouraging communication amongst primary care and other professionals in selected areas; and acting as a resource and focal point for encouraging primary care developments. The emphasis was on working with local practitioners not already in health centres and initially concentrating on practical problems in community health services. The project worker has also been meeting with GPs in health centres, encouraging them to think about the idea behind a health centre and emphasising the importance of teamwork. The setting up of GP liaison committees has provided the necessary support for GPs and consequently GP services are beginning to change. The project has also reviewed general practice services and produced maps showing the location of GP surgeries by size of practice and the location of women doctors.

The project is continuing to examine ways of providing practical support to GPs, for example the provision of an internal courier service to all GPs to enable quick delivery and collection of patients' notes and records and to encourage team communication and eliminate present heavy postal costs; assessing the feasibility of establishing a pathology courier service to GPs, to enable them to take and despatch specimens, thus reducing the resources needed for hospital staff to take specimens from patients; the provision of a regular information service to GPs about the availability and appropriate use of hospital and community services; and discussions with GPs about problems with patient groups, in particular, the highly mobile, the homeless, and ethnic minorities. This is done by arranging seminars and discussion groups for GPs and extending the availability of the interpreter service and liaison scheme to them. To overcome a lack of information on how to use services the project assisted the local CHC in the publication of a 'You and Your GP' leaflet, as well as GP lists and directories of open access clinic services.

In Camberwell a concrete and conscious response to Acheson was the Primary Medical Care Development Project which took up the Acheson suggestion that academic units of general practice might act to aid primary care development in inner cities. This project is based at the Department of General Practice Studies, King's College School of Medicine and Dentistry, and is being run by two GPs. However, this Department was not offered any Acheson money; the funding for the project is provided by the King's Fund. The aims of the project are: to improve contact with all general practitioners in the district in order to help them to identify their immediate and long-term service and educational needs, and consider possible solutions; to improve contact with the administration of community services and of the nursing and health visiting services, in order to increase liaison and attachment where possible and desired; to improve contact with those representing the point of view of patients and with academic and planning departments which can provide data to complement this; and to facilitate innovations within the individual practices or teams by providing information and discussion on the specific skills required to enable these developments to take place and to enable those with ideas or skills to share them. The overall concern of the project was thus to develop the ideas in the Acheson report. Unlike Dr Arnold Elliott's experimental project in Islington[12], the aim of this project is to develop primary care at a much more local level using immediate peers and colleagues, each of whom could offer knowledge, skills or expertise in particular fields useful to others in the district, on more of a self-help basis with all the advantages of continuity and flexibility.

The project set out to discover what GPs thought was important and to work from there. This apparently was the first time all local GPs had been offered a full opportunity to express their needs through individual discussion and thereby take part in planning future primary care services. The first task of the project was to make contact with GPs. This presented some difficulty as up-to-date lists of GPs were not available from the FPC. The project compiled its own lists from a variety of informal sources. It then undertook provision of information for GPs through improved communication and dialogue.

In Bloomsbury, one positive initiative following the publication of the Acheson report was the formation of a GPs' forum. The forum was established at the instigation of the Camden and Islington Local Medical Committee in October 1983. The initial reason for its formation was the fact that Bloomsbury Health Authority overlaps part of two areas—Camden and Islington and Kensington, Chelsea and Westminster—and it was proving difficult to respond to consultation documents from Bloomsbury because this involved getting together members representing parts of two LMCs. The forum, therefore, was intended to provide an informal meeting place for GPs in Bloomsbury. Its working aim is to promote co-operation between the district and the GPs working there, and all GPs practising with a main surgery in Bloomsbury are entitled to attend. The forum reports back to the two LMCs for ratification when any decision is taken and members of the Bloomsbury Health Authority Community Unit are invited to attend the meetings. GP attendance has been disappointing, however, and suggestions to improve attendance have been considered by the forum. The formation of the forum was welcomed by the district, however, as a way of facilitating close co-operation between the services provided by GPs and the Health Authority.

Initiatives to improve organisational arrangements
The organisational problems of primary health care as documented by the Acheson report were also heeded by the districts. Some set up specific mechanisms to discuss primary care, while others attempted to improve working relationships among primary health care workers. The City and Hackney DHA set up a steering group to guide the activities of the Primary Health Care Liaison Officer consisting of two GPs and the FPC administrator, as well as staff from community medicine, nursing, social services and the CHC. The appointment of the Primary Health Care Liaison Officer helped to catalyse developments, and to improve liaison among those involved in providing primary health care. It appears to have been an effective post because the officer was acceptable to community services, GPs, administrators and the FPC and understood how the system operated.

Unlike the City and Hackney Primary Care Liaison Officer, the Tower Hamlets Primary Care Project is not only funded by the King's Fund but is also independent of any department within the district. It is based at the Centre for the Study of Primary Care, which gives the development worker access to other staff at the Centre and helps liaison with the research activities of the Centre. Although there are obvious benefits in being independent and outside the mainstream structure, there are also disadvantages: the problem of isolation and difficulty in linking with many channels of communication. If not careful, the development worker can be viewed as an interferer rather than a facilitator. Furthermore, the work of the project has been hampered because of gaps in the administrative structure. At the moment there is no primary health care plannng team (there was one prior to 1981), and no-one with responsibility for future planning. There have also been some major changes in senior and middle management staffing which have further accentuated the fact that there is no planning structure. These factors have blunted the impact of the project. Nevertheless, senior and middle management have found the project useful and helpful. They feel that there is a need for a primary care development/facilitator officer as 'busy managers cannot do it all—you need someone to get things moving, particularly when there has been too much change in too short a space of time'. However, developments have been thwarted due to the lack of a planning structure and a number of steps have been taken to enable joint discussion and to improve procedures and communication. A GP Liaison Committee with hospital representatives has been established. Similarly a joint DHA and FPC Member Liaison Group has been formed. The function of this group is to exchange information and produce policy papers.

Camberwell District has a Primary Health Care Planning Team which consists of representatives from the Department of Community Medicine, the district medical officer, the specialist in community medicine, the senior health visitor, the senior nursing officer (community health), the FPC administrator, the treasurers, the unit administrator, the senior nurse planner, two GPs, two development officers of the two Social Services Departments, one member of the Community Health Council, the Information Officer and one member of the Primary Medical Care Development Project. This team has been considering primary care issues and the Acheson recommendations, and has also been involved in considering bids for the money made available following the report's publication. It has supervised the Primary Medical Care Development Project, encouraged joint training in teamwork among its own members, evaluated 'patch' and 'aligned' systems of community nurse deployment and supported the development of a Post-Graduate Medical Centre to improve training of GPs. Since the publication of the Acheson report, communication between hospitals and GPs has been better. The Accident and Emergency Departments have accepted that part of their work is about primary care. The new consultant concerned has liaised with the GPs and encouraged registration of patients.

Bloomsbury too has been developing good working arrangements with the two FPCs. The two FPC administrators meet the Community Unit Management Team each month at one of the regular meetings and share information and ideas and this enables them to establish better lines of communication. It is from these meetings that other issues are then taken up and discussed at formal and informal meetings.

Similarly, positive working relationships between the Victoria DHA and the FPCs were being developed and efforts were jointly being made to improve provision of primary care services.

Primary Health Care Teams
In accordance with the Acheson recommendations all the districts concerned are committed to the idea of attachments and teamwork, but progress on this front has been slow mainly because of practical problems like lack of suitable premises, inadequate multidisciplinary vocational training and the attitudes of those involved in primary care. Despite these difficulties attempts have been made to develop teamwork and attachments. For example, the Primary Care Liaison Officer in the City and Hackney DHA initially concentrated on meeting others involved in primary care, joining various co-ordinating and planning

groups and assessing problems relating to primary care. Interviews with GPs and nurses, discussions with those in nursing and community medicine and feedback to the planning groups helped to keep up the momentum on the question of attachments which perhaps would have been difficult without the post of Primary Care Liaison Officer. The district hopes to have district nurses attached to all practices before the end of 1985. Attachment of district nurses to general practices, however, has not been without difficulties. The nurses, for example, are experiencing varying amounts of difficulty in planning their visits because of the increased distances between patients and their unfamiliarity with areas of the district. To overcome these difficulties attached district nurses were provided with road maps and practices were encouraged to limit their catchment areas to a one-mile radius.

The Tower Hamlets DHA is also committed to attachments and to the concept of primary health care teams, but change is slow because of resistance from some GPs. However, the situation is developing as more younger, vocationally trained GPs are coming into the area. Moreover, the workload of the nursing staff is increasing because of high unemployment, child abuse and general deprivation. Shortage of staff has also affected progress on the question of attachments. Acheson monies have helped them to increase staff but problems of accommodation for the nursing staff and other necessary support remain.

The Primary Care Development Project has also been considering new approaches to planning primary care and through its link with the Centre for the Study of Primary Care consideration has been given to 'patchwork'.

The Camberwell Health District is gradually developing attachments but does not have a sufficient number of nurses to attach them to each practice. They have attempted instead to attach a nurse to a group of practices. On the whole the Acheson report has provided support to those in the nursing profession who were working towards the ideals contained in the report and has given some initiatives further impetus.

The Bloomsbury DHA recognises the difficulties which it faces in developing primary care teams but its strategy is nevertheless based on the Acheson recommendations. The aim is to serve Bloomsbury with a number of teams, each based in modern premises distributed throughout the district and sited centrally in the communities they serve. To this end a group of members of Bloomsbury's Community Unit Management Team in collaboration with the FPC hope to visit every GP in the district to determine the feasibility of these arrangements. The structure and composition of the teams would be flexible, and membership would be determined by the needs of the particular community served.

Similarly, the Victoria DHA has been attempting to improve and enhance primary health care services and encourage co-operation between GPs and community services. The relationship between the district and the FPC is good and collectively they are using a combination of tactics to bring about changes. The district is actively encouraging GP attachments and is thinking of making the question of attachments more explicit in the job descriptions. Lack of suitable GP premises remains a problem and a hindrance to developing attachments. Moreover, developing teamwork requires time and initiatives which can raise confidence and break down barriers.

Despite the difficulties which the districts face in developing teamwork, the Acheson money which was earmarked for training health visitors and district nurses did facilitate training of more nursing staff and to some extent helped to alleviate the problems caused by shortage of staff. In Camberwell, for example, the nursing services managed to train two health visitors and two district nurses in each of the first two years, and one health visitor and one district nurse in the third year. The Acheson money for training nursing staff proved to be the only way to recruit new staff in the present climate of economic stringency. This boost in staffing also helped with the development of attachments and teamwork, but these are affected by other underlying problems of small premises and single-handed practices. Acheson also created an opportunity for nurse managers to talk to doctors and provided an impetus for looking at alternative ways of working.

Improving GP premises
One of the problems alluded to in the Acheson report in relation to development of teamwork and attachments was the size and the quality of GP premises. Many of the GP premises in inner London are in poor condition or inadequate. Again in response to Acheson a number of steps have been taken by districts to improve the situation. The City and Hackney DHA, the FPC and the local authority have established a Premises Working Party whose main functions are to consider and co-ordinate the progress of applications for new or improved premises by GPs; to assist in drawing up areas of deficiency for expression in the borough plan; to prepare detailed guidance on the availability of funding and desirable standards of construction; to support and oversee the progress of application, through the council's procedures; and to develop a programme of improvement for GP premises. The working party meets every three weeks. Schemes which are put forward by GPs are considered and given the necessary support and help. The FPC is actively engaged in talking to GPs about cost-rent schemes and regularly visits GP premises. There is now a greater pressure by the FPC on the question of premises and it is prepared to suspend reimbursement if premises are not improved. It has been suggested that there is an evident change in the attitude of the FPC which now takes the view that it is there to administer the service. City and Hackney also appointed a GP accommodation visiting team some two years ago which carried out a survey of a limited number of premises. They involved the Medical Architecture Research Unit (MARU) of the Polytechnic of North London[13].

Similarly, in Tower Hamlets one of the main problems as far as GP services are concerned is the question of poor premises. Here the Primary Care Development Project arranged meetings with the Greater London Council, the FPC, the London borough of Tower Hamlets and MARU. Through these meetings some improvements have occurred and new methods of improving GP premises have been looked at. Prior to the project the GLC and the local authority were unaware that they were the major owners of GP premises in the district. Moreover, the improvement grant scheme had not been made use of in the district. In the summer of 1984 the FPC and the Health Authority published a paper suggesting guidelines for the development of primary care premises, which were supported by the local council[14]. Now a joint working group with the London borough of Tower Hamlets is being established to encourage the review and improvement or replacement of inadequate GP premises.

Improvements are evidently taking place in those areas where the DHAs, FPCs and local authorities are collaborating to bring about change. In Camberwell, however, there was criticism that the FPC did not stimulate GPs to take up the increased improvement grants. The take-up, therefore, has been rather uneven. On the other hand, in Bloomsbury in order to improve GP premises the District Management Team (DMT) allocated a notional sum of £100,000 to be made available from its 'pump-priming' sources. This was money which was expected to become available from reducing activity in the acute sector as a result of specifically formulated and previously agreed plans. At the same time the GP Forum was asked to identify how this money could be used and by what practices.

The strategic impact of Acheson

What is evident from these developments is that the Acheson report not only reinforced the ideas which were already in currency and provided greater impetus for change, but also influenced the future priorities of districts. City and Hackney Health Authority's Strategic Plan 1983-93 made reference to the organisational problems of general practice as documented by the Acheson report and proposed further development of primary health care teams along with patch-based care and closer liaison between the community health services and general practitioners. Against this background the DHA has made progress on several grants, including the change in the use of St Leonard's Hospital, which will provide a base for the Community Unit and Community Nursing Service, with its main function being to provide an integrated out-patient facility with open access to GPs. Discussions are also taking place about the development of a University GP practice which will take on the responsibility of providing medical cover for the walk-in treatment centre, and extend the range of facilities available to registered and non-registered patients, particularly the homeless and rootless.

In view of the high level of deprivation, several approaches have been used in Tower Hamlets to develop a more effective primary care service. Initiatives include five new health centres in areas of great need where GP and clinic premises were totally inadequate; and the provision of a new clinic on the Isle of Dogs to meet the needs of the growing population. The district is also aiming to provide support to families and young children. It has appointed health visitors who speak Bengali and six interpreters to assist at health clinics and/or home visits. Health visitors are attached to GPs who have suitable accommodation.

The district has established a strong community and psychiatric unit of management and has obtained King's Fund finance for a three-year Mental Health Initiative Project in order to encourage the development of community psychiatric and psychology services. It has also developed three well-woman clinics to provide a full screening service for women whose GPs are not providing such a service or who may want advice from women staff. Close liaison and support of the Maternity Services Liaison Scheme which provides a service to non-English-speaking women to help them use maternity services have been developed. Similarly other community support schemes are being developed to enable patients to be cared for at home where possible. Acheson and inner city funds have been used to establish a night nursing scheme and a family aid service.

The presence of the Centre for the Study of Primary Care has encouraged action-orientated research. Studies looking at 'inappropriate' use of hospital accident and emergency services and discussion of new procedures to encourage patients to use appropriate primary care services have been encouraged. Primary health care staff generally feel the benefit of this Centre, as they can attend seminars, and make contact with others.

Camberwell DHA's Strategic Plan for 1985-94 takes full cognisance of national and regional policies in the field of primary care and sees the main future issues in Camberwell as being the need to develop provision for neighbourhoods and groups which are underserved by health facilities; better organisational arrangements for providing services; greater sensitivity on the part of professional staff to the health needs and expectations of diverse communities; better access to GPs; and multidisciplinary training which will assist mutual understanding of roles and relationships between members of primary health care teams.

Accordingly, the district's programme for 1984-94 aims to support the development of a post-graduate Medical Centre to enable greater integration between GPs and hospital medical staff and improve communication between the hospital and primary health care teams. The programme also examines the present distribution and management of clinic facilities to improve access and take-up of services. The district aims to work with the FPC and other interested agencies to encourage GPs to accept the attachment of health care workers and the take-up of grants to upgrade premises; to increase numbers in community nursing; to develop community information services to examine linkages between social factors and health care and provide a system of early diagnosis; to promote strategies which raise levels of public knowledge about health care issues and involve local people in defining their own health needs; and to assess the changes in service provision which are needed to meet the health needs of the ethnic communities living within the boundaries of the district.

Following the 1982 reorganisation the District Management Team of the Victoria DHA conceived the need for a district strategy, and as an initial task compiled the relevant information and developed a statistical modelling technique for the projection of service requirements. This report was published in June 1983[15]. The second report which moved on to the analysis of possible strategies was published in August 1984[16]. This document put the whole ques-

Table 4.2   Allocation of Acheson money

(i)   *City and Hackney DHA*

Acheson money 1983/84 for primary care projects	£
Premises—Health Centres improvements in accommodation	3,500
District Nursing services nursing aids and equipment	2,700
Miscellaneous accommodation for social worker in clinic	2,000
Health visiting services mobile clinic (child health and well woman clinic services)	9,700
Health visiting services nursing equipment	3,200
Night nursing services—car	4,000
School health services—typewriter	2,000
Total allocation	27,000

(ii)   *Tower Hamlets DHA*

Acheson money 1983/84 for primary care projects	£
Incontinence project Centre for the Study of Primary Care	2,300

Acheson money 1984/85 for primary care projects	
Teamwork facilitator Centre for the Study of Primary Care	14,000
District nurse training	9,600
Total allocation	23,600

Acheson money 1985/86 for primary care projects	
Health promotion (video equipment)	66,000
Teamwork facilitator	14,000
Total allocation	80,000

(iii)   *Camberwell DHA*

Acheson money 1983/84 for primary care projects	£
Research Project	4,500
Social deprivation/Health	

Information Systems	
Acorn mapping	1,500
Computer hardware	6,000
Street maps	1,000
Extension of Whaddon House clinic	8,000
Community zoning plan including condition survey/valuation of premises	3,000
Car for health visitor use	7,000
Total allocation in 1983/84	31,000

Table 4.2 Allocation of Acheson money (continued)

Acheson money 1984/85 for primary care projects
physiological measurement technician   12,000

(iv) *Bloomsbury DHA*

Acheson money 1983/84 for primary care projects	£
Crown car	5,000
3 electric beds	3,000
Total allocation	8,000

Acheson money 1984/85 for primary care projects	£
Car	3,000
General expenses	2,000
Health visitor salary (travelling facilities)	3,000
Health visitor salary (travelling facilities)	3,000
Total allocation	11,000

(v) *Victoria DHA*

Acheson money 1983/84 for primary care projects	£
Advertising in Yellow Pages re-registration with GPs	5,500
Women's health catalogue	3,000
Antenatal booklets	2,000
Revised antenatal booklets	5,000
Survey of medical needs in hostels for the homeless	3,000
Follow up of Accident and Emergency patients not registered with a GP	3,300
Total allocation	21,500

Acheson money 1984/85 for primary care projects	
Identifying patients registering with GPs following visits to Accident and Emergency departments	1,800
Support in establishing age-sex registers	1,000
Computer software for existing registers	2,000
Total allocation	4,800

Acheson money 1985/86 for primary health care projects	
Support in establishing age-sex registers	3,320
Night nursing system for 20 elderly patients	17,400
Pilot study to prepare a detailed programme of medical needs which could be implemented by the DHA and FPC	3,000
Total allocation	23,720

tion of health care in the community into a broader context. It stated that the founding hopes of the National Health Service, namely, that easier access to health care would diminish sickness and lead to a decline in demand on services, was mistaken; secondly, that the revolution in biomedical sciences had led to a concentration of resources in the acute sector of the health service, 'cure' as opposed to 'care' services; thirdly, that the underlying philosophy of medical care was wrong, and that the resources devoted to medical research merely indicated that it was costing more to achieve no more in terms of quality of life for patients; and finally that an effective comprehensive health care system cannot be achieved without due regard for the socioeconomic environment in which it takes place. It argued that health care cannot be isolated from its social context and that the financial restraints on the economy have ensured that primary health care is at the forefront of these issues. The development of a strategy for health care in the community, therefore, has to be set in this context, and the issues for consideration in Victoria are to be based on four principles: objective measures of need, demonstrable cost-effectiveness, social benefit and the relationship of health services to primary care.

The report spelt out the rationale for increased resources to be allocated to selected primary care services, and for reassessment of the role played by hospital accident and emergency departments. It stated:

since access to general medical services is difficult in inner cities—the reasons for which are pin-pointed in the Acheson Report, and are not susceptible to the influence of the DHA or the FPC—then the corresponding demands made by patients on hospitals should be recognised, and hospital Accident and Emergency departments appropriately staffed to take an *explicit* part in the pattern of primary care[17].

Against these broad analyses Victoria Health Authority developed short-term proposals for primary health care for 1984/85, 1985/86 and 1986/87. These included a detailed profile of the community served by Victoria, and proposals for a health centre policy, family planning services, services for the homeless, night nursing services, and support services for cases in the community. To implement these short-term proposals Victoria used the Acheson money for a number of projects. A survey was undertaken to assess the extent to which accident and emergency facilities were being used where a consultation with a general practitioner might be more appropriate, and to identify patients who register with GPs following visits to the Accident and Emergency department. Secondly, a survey of local GPs suggested that doctors are interested in establishing age/sex registers. This record system is invaluable in identifying groups at particular risk and those requiring screening and immunisation and is an important tool in preventive medicine. Thirdly, a project was established to provide a night nursing and sitting service with the aim of employing suitable people to sit with the elderly and frail at night so as to give normal 'family' care throughout the night. Finally, some money was used for clinical facilities and equipment for improved medical and nursing services in hostels for the single homeless. This need was identified following a survey of the health needs of the single homeless in hostels.

Family Practitioner Committees

The Acheson report made substantial criticisms of the Family Practitioner Committees and of the ways in which they arrange the provision of services. A brief look at three FPCs, namely City and East London, Lambeth, Southwark and Lewisham, and the Kensington and Chelsea and Westminster, which cover the five districts discussed earlier, suggests that in some areas FPCs have become more active and are beginning to take positive initiatives in planning.

The City and East London FPC, which covers City and Hackney, Tower Hamlets and Newham Health Authorities, has been taking initiatives to appoint GPs who are committed to teamwork. On the question of GP premises the FPC has been talking to doctors about cost-rent schemes, has appointed a GP accommodation team, has been visiting premises and working jointly with the respective health districts and local authorities to improve premises, and has collaborated with health authorities in order to develop GP services. Because the FPC was active and taking the necessary initiatives the demand for improvement grants was enormous, and the FPC used all the extra money which was made available by the DHSS. Since the appointment of the Primary Health Care Liaison Officer in City and Hackney Health Authority, the FPC has been involved in the planning stages of the relevant initiatives.

The administrator of the Lambeth, Southwark and Lewisham Family Practitioner Committee which covers Camberwell Health District argued that the criticisms contained in the Acheson report did not apply to his FPC because its circumstances were closer to those of outer London boroughs than inner London boroughs. Unlike Tower Hamlets and City and Hackney, the area covered by the Lambeth, Southwark and Lewisham FPC has good residential districts where GPs live, so that they are accessible. The area, it was stated, has enough group practices; moreover, it was pointed out that there is evidence to show that group practices have a high turnover of patients because patients do not like the appointment system or seeing different doctors. Furthermore, there are practical problems in encouraging group practices since there are not enough large premises. It was suggested that any change in that direction would be slow. For example, in the last few years only one practice had qualified for additional allowance, and that was a health centre which has been in gestation for fifteen years. The change, therefore, was not stimulated by the new group practice allowance. Improvement grants, on the other hand, have yielded some benefits. Five surgeries had improved their premises.

On the question of encouraging young doctors, it was said that there was an over-supply of young doctors and that there were no realistic vacancies for them. Moreover, older doctors had an advantage of seniority, and if one was seeking to do the best for patients and aiming to provide a good family doctor service then seniority and experience were an advantage.

The Kensington and Chelsea and Westminster FPC, which covers the Victoria Health Authority, took a number of steps in response to Acheson.

First, it organised routine visits to surgeries and those which were found to be unsatisfactory were brought to the attention of the FPC. Second, at the request of the FPC, the North West Thames RHA agreed to appoint a coordinator/facilitator for the FPC area. Third, all new doctors in primary care are reminded to contact the FPC if they need temporary residential accommodation. Fourth, the FPC has reminded and advised all GPs about making suitable arrangements for telephone cover. Fifth, GPs have been asked to display information regarding the use of answering machines, and information about call interceptors has been collected by the FPC and is available to patients on request. Sixth, whenever practice arrangements are discussed with GPs, they are encouraged to concentrate their practice areas so as to facilitate close working relationships with other primary care workers.

Recently, the Kensington and Chelsea and Westminster FPC appointed a development officer whose main responsibility is to continue with the implementation of the Acheson recommendations, and under the new arrangements for FPCs[18] work out a five-year strategy and prepare an annual report. The development officer is also required to decide upon the approach to issues and problems, highlight deficiencies in the service, act as a catalyst and develop consultation mechanisms. New arrangements provide a new opportunity for a planning role which, until recently, was non-existent. Under this new impetus, Kensington, Chelsea and Westminster FPC plans to look at issues such as attachments, deficiencies in the service, emergency dental service, provision for ethnic minorities, drug misuse and direct consultation with groups and neighbours.

The FPC is also involved with the Victoria Health Authority in a working party on primary health care and has a good rapport with the district. They are planning to advertise GP services in the 'Yellow Pages' and this initiative will be funded by Acheson money. The FPC has continued to inspect GP premises and has encouraged applications for improvement grants and cost-rent schemes on which it has also produced guidance notes. If GPs have any problems regarding planning permission they are encouraged to contact the FPC for relevant assistance. On the question of encouraging younger GPs, the Medical Vacancies Committee considered the Acheson recommendations and came to the conclusion that it was duty-bound to consider all applicants. However, recently four out of five vacancies have been filled by younger doctors.

A brief look at these three FPCs illustrates the fact that, apart from the powers which FPCs have, a great deal depends upon the administrator and how he or she interprets the job. The new status of family practitioner committees as autonomous authorities provides more and not less opportunity for FPCs to plan their services and play a more strategic role in association with health authorities and local authorities in providing effective primary health care. If FPCs are committed to the ideals of Acheson then reorganisation is a new opportunity.

Summing up

A look at three regions, five district health authorities and three FPCs shows that changes, some concrete and others less so, are taking place locally. Emphases and responses vary but it is clear that the Acheson report and a limited amount of extra money provided a gentle push for health authorities, FPCs and others. The report was found to be a useful background and reference document for those trying to promote primary care. Moreover, the thinking and the ideas contained in the Acheson report are now part of conventional wisdom.

The main concern at the local level centres on how best to implement the necessary changes. Local managers and administrators have had to cope with too much change in a fairly short space of time. Effecting change not only requires time, energy and staff resources but also shifts in priorities and resources. At a time when resources are scarce and the emphasis is on diverting resources from one sector of the health service to another, then a question of the realism of this expectation arises. Secondly, changes such as developing primary health care teams or new patterns of working relationships, changes in the attitudes of GPs and nurses, and establishing effective administrative and organisational mechanisms for planning and delivering primary care services will take time.

Despite the constraints and obstacles Acheson gave impetus to certain ideas and the Report, taken together with limited financial incentives, has led to some significant changes. The area where the extra money appears to have had some effect is in the field of training of nurses. Extra money has enabled districts to boost their nursing staff complement or maintain an adequate level of staff. This in turn has, to a limited extent, helped the districts to implement some changes in their working arrangements. On the question of GP premises some FPCs, in response to the criticism voiced in the Acheson report, have encouraged GPs to make use of cost-rent schemes and improvement grants. The criticism also led to joint initiatives by FPCs, local authorities and district health authorities. For example, Tower Hamlets and City and Hackney with their FPC invited the Medical Architecture Research Unit, based at the North London Polytechnic, to look at the stock of GP premises and advise on developments. Similarly, initiatives such as the appointment of a Primary Care Liaison Worker in City and Hackney and the establishment of Primary Care Development Projects in Tower Hamlets and Camberwell have assisted better liaison, helped to establish mechanisms for better co-ordination and helped to involve FPCs in the planning process.

These projects are essentially filling a real need in bringing people together (particularly GPs, who previously have been working in isolation) and drawing them into the planning process. This has helped to change attitudes and assist change. The Departments of General Practice too have taken a more active role, and the establishment of primary health care planning teams and other administrative arrangements between districts and FPCs have contributed positively to developments. The problems of providing effective primary care services as outlined in the Acheson report remain, but on the whole the report has had a positive effect at local level and has assisted the process of change.

References

1   *Primary Health Care in Inner London*, Report of a study group commissioned by the London Health Planning Consortium, May 1981, para.1.18.
2   *Survey of Primary Care in London*, Report of a Working Party of the RCGP, May 1981.
3   *Inequalities in Health*, Report of a research working group, DHSS, 1980.
4   North East Thames Regional Health Authority, *Planning for primary care: a discussion document*, 1978. Hackney/Islington Inner City Partnership, *Report of primary health care (Hackney) sub-group*, 1979. *Report of primary health care (Islington) sub-group*, 1979.
5   The Centre for the Study of Primary Care based at the Steels Lane Health Centre, London Borough of Tower Hamlets. The centre was formally opened on 28 April 1983.
6   Members' Panel on Primary Care Report to the South East Thames Regional Health Authority, February 1984 (Draft 3).
7   South East Thames Regional Health Authority, *Outline Regional Strategy: 1985-1994*, Section 5.9, Primary Care Services.
8   North West Thames Regional Health Authority, *Regional Strategy. Towards a strategy for primary health care*, September 1984.
9   *Ibid.*, para.4.1.
10 *The Brixton Disorders, 10-12 April 1981.* A report by the Rt Hon. The Lord Scarman, OBE, HMSO, 1981.
11 North East Thames Regional Health Authority, *Planning for Primary Care: a discussion document, 1978.* Report of Primary Health Care (Hackney) sub-group, 1979.
12 Arnold Elliott, 'General practice facilitator—a personal view', *Health Trends*, vol. 16, no.4, November 1984, pp.74-79.
13 The Medical Architecture Research Unit (MARU), of the Polytechnic of North London, is a multi-disciplinary unit which carries out research and consultancy on the planning, design and evaluation of health buildings. Inner London Primary Health Care Practice Premises Unit was established in 1982 by the King's Fund within MARU. From 1984 the work of the unit is being supported by funding from the DHSS.
14 *Primary Care in Tower Hamlets—future policy and liaison in provision of General Practitioner Premises*, Tower Hamlets Health Authority and the City and East London FPC, 1984.
15 *Evaluation of Health Services in Victoria: A Strategic Framework for the Future*, Vol. I, Victoria Health Authority, June 1983.
16 *Evaluation of Health Services in Victoria: A Strategic Framework for the Future*, Vol. II, Victoria Health Authority, August 1984.
17 *Ibid.*, Section 6, para.6(d), p.72.
18 The Report of the Joint Working Group on Collaboration between Family Practitioner Committees and District Health Authorities, April 1984.

CHAPTER 5   THE ACHESON REPORT AND AFTER

Introduction

Detailed examination of the origin of a committee of inquiry and of the subsequent fate of its report, such as has been attempted in the preceding chapters, might seem to lead naturally to the question 'what difference has it made?' In the case of the Acheson inquiry the question would be in the form 'what effect has the Acheson report had on the provision of primary health care services in inner London?'

A pragmatic approach of this kind with its emphasis on outcomes may seem not only the most appropriate way of reaching a conclusion, but entirely in keeping with the assumed rationality of appointing committees of inquiry in the first place. How else can one justify bringing together a group of eminent and busy people to toil for months over intractable problems, if the object is not to make some significant impact on those problems?

The question of what effect Acheson has had is indeed important, but it is not easy to give a direct answer to it. Partly, this is a matter of practical limitations. While Acheson money is still being used and projects funded by it are fairly new, it is difficult to make a comprehensive assessment of its practical consequences. Moreover, any assessment must take account of the fact that changes in this field are bound to be slow. A further general difficulty is that it is not easy to isolate the influence of committees of inquiry. The fact, for example, that there are more younger doctors practising in inner London than there were when the Acheson committee began work raises the question of how far this is attributable to the influence of the committee's report and how far to other factors.

More generally, as has been pointed out elsewhere[1], committees of inquiry are not isolated phenomena appearing out of the blue, but elements in a continuing process of evolution of policy, and the part which any individual committee can play depends very much on its relationship to all the other factors which are shaping that policy. And clearly one important element here is not only the precise recommendations which a committee makes but the extent to which its analysis affects the ideas and attitudes of others participating in the policy process.

It is for this reason that previous chapters have emphasised not only the immediate context within which the Acheson committee was appointed and operated but also the wider issues and events which are relevant to an understanding of the part which it played in the field of primary health care policy.

In this final chapter, therefore, we do not attempt to answer directly the question of what difference the Acheson report has made to the provision of primary health care in inner London. Instead, we examine two related matters: the nature and adequacy of the response to the problems analysed and discussed in the Acheson report; and the possibilities of future progress in dealing with those problems. Such an approach depends on certain assumptions both about the nature of the problems and, more broadly, about the ways in which policy is developed within the NHS, and these assumptions will be made explicit in the course of the discussion.

In adopting this approach, we are conscious that it leaves many questions unanswered about the adequate provision of primary health care services in London. Indeed, given the importance of the subject, further work needs to be done to elucidate the extent to which progress has been made in improving that provision and the factors which contribute to and hinder progress, with a view to identifying the direction which future policy and practice should follow. The present study may therefore be regarded as a preliminary investigation on which further research may build.

We first draw attention to one major theme which is critical for the whole study and has frequently been alluded to in previous chapters. We have referred above to the Acheson report as though it has relevance only for London. But in fact two sets of problems need to be kept in mind: the particular problems of London, and the general problems of inner cities. Earlier chapters have shown how the two became inextricably intertwined especially in terms of the reaction of central government to the Acheson report. The essence of the matter is that the provision of primary health care services in the inner cities was a problem field well before the Acheson inquiry was instituted and that no effective response to it had been made in terms of national policies and priorities. London had its own distinctive problems which were brought to a head by proposals to reduce the acute bed provision in inner London and these provided the immediate occasion for the appointment of the Acheson committee.

Although the relationship between these two sets of problems was not made clear at the time when the committee was appointed, there can be no doubt that the way in which it approached its task, the depth of its analysis and the range of its recommendations ensured that any national policy response could not be confined to London. The idea of putting forward immediate short-term measures deriving from existing studies to meet the specific needs of London was in any case overlaid by the need to seek a wider view, as the DHSS's letter of December 1979 to Professor Acheson made clear. It was unrealistic to suppose that such a wider view would not have exposed some general issues affecting other inner cities even if the committee had interpreted its terms of reference more narrowly than it did.

From the point of view of the present analysis the situation poses some difficulties. The national policy response to the Acheson report was not confined to London, but applied to all those inner city areas where partnership and programme arrangements had been agreed. Discussion of government response to the report must therefore take this into account and must indeed be critically concerned with the reasons why a report which considered only London's problems became the basis of measures to improve primary health care in the inner cities generally. On the other hand, the fact that the Acheson analysis was strictly confined to the situation as the committee found it in London makes it sensible to study the response at the local level in London alone. This is what has been done here, but it must be borne in mind that it by no means follows that authorities in other inner city areas have reacted in quite the same way either to the report or to the 'Acheson money' offered by the government.

The response to the Acheson report

To ask whether the response to a committeee report has been adequate presupposes a certain view of the nature of the report itself. It assumes in fact that action along the lines recommended was desirable. Was this true of the Acheson report? In this study the view has been taken that the analysis of deficiencies in the provision of primary health care in inner London was on conventional lines, and that the committee looked for remedies which could be applied within the existing structure of the NHS. In other words, it was not looking to some totally new approach to solve the problems of primary health care. Nor did its proposals threaten any existing established interests in the NHS. A possible exception to this statement is the proposal for a retirement policy for GPs which might be taken as a threat to their independent contractor status. It is, however, possible, as some GPs at least recognise, to combine the two, and despite the opposition to the Acheson proposal it is difficult to regard it as in any sense a subversive or indeed particularly radical proposal.

Within its self-imposed limits the committee provided in fact a set of sensible and practical proposals. This is to take an overall view. It does not mean that every proposal was likely to be equally effective, nor does it mean that the committee's assessment of the likely consequences of adopting a proposal has in every case to be accepted. These are all matters for debate and can give rise to significant disagreement. But what does seem evident is that, taken as a whole, the committee's proposals could have made a marked impact on the problems of primary health care in inner London, and, by implication, in other inner cities too. To a large extent this is because the underlying thrust of the report is towards the necessity for shifting more resources into primary health care. What the report does in addition is to specify those areas where the impact ought, if the committee is right, to be most pronounced. Again, to say this is to say nothing about whether the committee produced the 'right' report. To do that would require a more profound analysis dealing with such questions as whether 'solving' the problems of primary health care in inner cities requires a more radical approach, discarding the assumptions and self-imposed limitations of the committee. All that is being claimed here is that if the committee's recommendations had been acted on and pursued with vigour they would have made some impression on the problems identified in its analysis.

However, neither at national nor at local level has the major shift in priorities and resources towards primary health care which the Acheson report called for taken place in practice. Nationally, some additional resources were provided but, apart from the fact that they did not cover some important areas identified by Acheson (for example, financial incentives to GPs to register new patients), they have been inadequate to provide a sustained shift in priorities towards primary care in the inner cities. Nor, apart from commending the Acheson report to health and other authorities, has the centre done much to ensure that that shift takes place at local level. Indeed, the evidence from London presented in this study indicates that any expectation that such a shift might take places has proved unrealistic, and what has been revealed is a mismatch between strategic thinking and operational planning.

Nor is it only a question of the total of resources provided. So far as the government's measures are concerned, the purposes for which those resources were allocated and the nature of the government's commitment which they revealed are also important. The main characteristics of those measures may be summed up as:

i)   they constitute a piecemeal, unco-ordinated approach to the problems of primary health care in the inner cities;

ii) they represent a short-term approach, a temporary stimulus rather than a continuing commitment.

Taken together, these assertions amount to saying that the government response was inadequate and did not match the needs identified by the Acheson report so far as London was concerned and as subsequently applied to the inner cities generally. This is a severe indictment which must be justified before considering the reasons for this inadequate response.

Whatever may have been the original intention of the DHSS in negotiating with the professions on the Acheson proposals, what emerged was a £9m package which consisted partly of measures deriving more or less directly from Acheson recommendations and partly of other measures not suggested by Acheson. There is no indication that this precise set of measures was chosen because it made sense in terms of the Acheson analysis, or even that it made the best use of the available money, nor was it justified in these terms. Government spokesmen merely claimed that the measures would contribute to the improvement of primary health care in inner cities and were part of a continuing effort to give priority to this area of health care.

Yet a critical question is surely: if primary health care in the inner cities is to have priority, should there not be some indication of how these measures fit into an overall strategy, and, in particular, how measures mainly limited to a three-year period can be expected to have longer-term consequences? For the message of the Acheson report is that if we are serious about wanting to improve primary health care in inner London then there must be a permanent shift of resources in that direction.

Three things might be said in answer to these points. In the first place, it is unrealistic to expect committee reports to be accepted in toto and, therefore, some selection of recommendations is inevitable. There is clearly much force in this argument. On the other hand, where recommendations are rejected or modified in favour of some rather different set of proposals, it is not perhaps unreasonable to expect that the new proposals should relate to an identifiable objective. Instead, what was offered by Acheson as a wide-ranging series of recommendations which could, taken together, make a significant attempt to deal with longstanding problems has been turned into a disjointed set of measures whose only common feature is that each of them individually can be said to do something towards improving, even if only temporarily, the provision of primary health care in the inner cities.

Secondly, it could be said that the committee itself did not help by ignoring the invitation to indicate priorities for action, so that there is no guide to what in the committee's view would be most worth doing if it were not possible to do everything it recommended. Given the composition of the committee and the scope of the investigations which it decided to undertake, it would have been impossible in practice for it to have arrived at a precise view of priorities. Nevertheless, as was discussed in an earlier chapter, it is possible to discern some real but undisclosed priorities from a close reading of the report. A more important point is, however, that it is difficult to believe that the nature of the government's response to the Acheson report had much to do with the failure to indicate priorities. The nature of the committee's report, although undoubtedly a factor, was not the major influence on the government's response.

The third argument which might be used to justify the rather limited response made by the government is that the main responsibility for ensuring priority for inner city primary health care lies with the authorities operating locally. This is an argument, however, which requires rather more careful examination than merely pointing to the fact that many recommendations in the Acheson report were directed at these authorities and not at central government. Of course, recommendations such as that district nurses should have access to social and recreational facilities provided for hospital staff are entirely a matter for district health authorities, but what we should be more concerned about here is the nature of the response by authorities operating locally, and its relationship to the national response.

Here one can distinguish two main elements in the local response, as was indicated in the previous chapter on the basis of what was happening in London. In the first place, the Acheson report, because it gave authoritative backing to ideas which were already around but needed to be implemented, proved useful to those trying to promote developments in primary care. They could draw on it and use it to strengthen the argument for introducing new measures or modifying old ones. Secondly, there was the positive incentive provided by Acheson money. Authorities naturally varied in the nature and emphasis of their response, but the very fact of bidding for resources concentrated the minds of those planning services and encouraged thinking on how best to utilise extra resources. Each district used the money according to its perceived needs.

Two examples may be given of the positive stimulus provided by Acheson money and the Acheson report. Extra money for training of nurses has enabled districts to boost their nursing staff complement or maintain an adequate level of staff. This in turn has helped districts to implement some changes in their working arrangements. The fact that the money was limited and for a short period means that the impact too will be limited. In the short term, however, the districts have benefited and have been able to implement some changes whose effect may be long-lasting.

In London at least, therefore, the Acheson report and the limited amount of money which has been made available have provided a gentle push for health authorities, FPCs and others. Changes have been taking place which are in keeping with Acheson ideas. But the fact that much of this has been in response to money made available by central government illustrates the interdependence of national and local policies. The argument that many of the Acheson recommendations were directed specifically at health authorities and family practitioner committees should not be considered in isolation. It is the total combined response which is important. Central government's response is important mainly in two ways which in turn affect the local response: directly, in the resources it makes available; indirectly, in that the perceived importance to central government of improving primary health care in the inner cities may help to influence the attitudes of local policy-makers.

One other point arises here. A major part of the government's response to the Acheson report, as measured by the amount of money allocated to it, was not in fact related to the report's recommendations but called for 'innovative ideas' from health authorities. That may be seen as part of a stimulus from central government to local initiative. But whatever the value of individual projects funded in this way, the very inclusion of this approach in a package of measures designed to further the aims of the Acheson report in fact draws attention to the gulf between them. There are arguments for stimulating local initiatives to improve primary health care, but they have little to do with the Acheson analysis. They could have been put forward at any time without carrying out a detailed examination of the problems. This is very different from devising a set of measures which make sense as a whole and as part of a general plan. There is no guarantee that several hundred individual projects, however worthy each may be, approved under the very general criterion of being 'of immediate benefit to primary health care services', will in total prove an effective way of channelling increased resources into the primary health care sector, particularly given the difficulties of sustaining many projects once the initial funding has ceased.

The innovative ideas measure in particular is an indication of the true nature of the package announced in October 1983. It was to show that something was being done to improve the provision of primary health care in the inner cities, and the coherence of the package was less important than the need to put together something workable within a limited and temporary budget. But if there are any lessons for the future to be learned from this study of the Acheson report it is necessary to make clear why the government response took the form it did.

In considering this question it is hard to avoid the conclusion that practically everything was against either a swift or a substantial response to the Acheson report. The most prominent factors were of a general nature, especially the political and economic situation, but there were in addition more specific factors directly related to the Acheson inquiry, and to the nature of policy-making in the NHS.

Undoubtedly, the main obstacles to a more positive response to the Acheson report lay in the political and economic circumstances which have prevailed since 1979. The Labour government of 1974-79 may have failed to take up the challenge of primary health care in the inner cities, but at least inner city problems generally had a degree of priority even at a time of severe economic constraints. The main priority for the Conservative government elected in 1979, however, was the attack on inflation with its concomitant emphasis on the reduction of public expenditure. Existing policies and commitments were scrutinised in this light, not least the inner city policy initiated by the Labour government in 1977. In the circumstances, primary health care in the inner cities would have needed a much higher priority than the government was prepared to give it if there was to be any chance of attracting additional resources on the scale seen as necessary by the Acheson committee.

The detailed consequences have been discussed earlier, both in the long delays which occurred before the government made its response, and in the nature of the package of measures which eventually emerged. The latter was, however, further shaped by some of the more specific factors referred to above. In particular, unwillingness to go directly against views strongly held by the professions and more especially the medical profession, which is a general characteristic of policy-making in the NHS, contributed to the further whittling down of the Acheson proposals. The fact that a report concerned only with inner London had implications for the inner cities generally is also relevant here, since the BMA in particular was strongly opposed to action being taken in relation to London alone. Thus there was the further difficulty of finding a way of applying the Acheson proposals to the inner cities generally, with consequent financial implications among others. Again, the fact that the report was so wide-ranging and contained a good many proposals which had longer-term implications made its acceptance politically more difficult than if it had been more limited and short-term. Finally, it must be noted that the administrative structure of the NHS makes for difficulties in devising and carrying out effective strategies for primary health care. A major obstacle to planning is the division between services provided by health authorities on the one hand and family practitioner committees on the other, and this accentuated the difficulties of carrying through a policy directed at a limited target like the inner cities.

Together, these constituted formidable obstacles. On the other side, there was little beyond the fact that primary health care in the inner cities was a nagging problem, on which the medical profession in particular had maintained pressure for a number of years. Whether this would have been sufficient to have evoked a response to Acheson without the fortuitous intervention of the inner city riots of 1981 is uncertain. But it seems clear that from some time in 1981 the government was committed to doing something about the problems of primary health care in the inner cities.

In the circumstances it is not surprising that what emerged was not a coherent plan deriving from the Acheson report but rather a series of measures which could be introduced relatively easily and which did not have major implications for public expenditure. Measured against the needs as identified by Acheson for London and by implication for other inner cities, the response was inadequate. Measured against the political and economic pressures in particular, it is perhaps surprising that even this much was achieved.

Above all, the response to the Acheson report exemplifies a general feature of social policy, namely that, except under very favourable conditions, the pace of change is slow. Those who seized on the report in expectation of a swift and favourable response from government were therefore bound to be disappointed.

After Acheson

So far we have been concerned with describing and analysing what has happened following the Acheson report. But a major concern now must be to see what lessons can be derived from this account for the future. We therefore now turn to an examination of questions which need to be answered if health authorities and FPCs are to operate more effectively to further the development of primary health care in the inner cities, and what part the DHSS might play in stimulating that development.

One set of questions concerns the role of the regions. There is, first, a problem which specifically affects only London. In providing money for primary care projects, the DHSS used the existing channels for allocating money, that is, regions were asked to bid for sums stated.

Was this the most effective way of allocating resources? Should the DHSS have encouraged more strategic use of the money by encouraging the regions to collaborate on issues such as 'setting up of a team of co-ordinators for inner London to liaise with responsible bodies and build up a profile of land available in areas of need, help GPs in searching for suitable premises and promote groupings of practices', as suggested by Acheson? Some argue that inner London is a special case (reasons for this are well rehearsed), and requires a co-ordinated approach. Territorial division of inner London into four regions not only increases the possibility of duplication of effort but also blunts and dissipates the impact of resources. Co-ordination on the question of GP premises perhaps would have improved communication between different parties and allowed for professional input. The question which, in future, needs further consideration is whether some initiatives should be taken jointly by the regions and what role the DHSS should play in encouraging this. There is perhaps a need for a two-pronged approach, that is, funding which encourages collaboration by London regions, and funding for local initiatives which is used to develop projects in response to local needs.

A more general question regarding the role of the regions arises from the way in which they distributed the available money between different categories. The four Thames regions showed considerable variety in the criteria they adopted for this purpose. Admittedly, it is not easy for regions to respond quickly to small packages of money, and it is perhaps difficult to justify a great deal of involvement in decisions on such modest sums of money. But should the regions have frameworks which are robust and flexible enough to facilitate effective allocation of small packages of extra resources? This question needs to be considered against the overall function of regions. Apart from allocation of resources to DHAs, the regions are responsible for long-term strategic policies and plans, stretching ten years ahead, for major building projects, medical education and manpower planning. Given these functions, what should be the role of regions in the development of effective primary health care provision? Secondly, given the administrative structure of the NHS (that is, independence of FPCs and the fact that most FPC boundaries do not match DHA boundaries, while in parts FPCs also overlap regional boundaries), what impact can regions have on so many tiers of the NHS? What the regions have is the potential for co-ordinating different facets of the NHS and, through this co-ordination, developing planning systems which can facilitate better allocation of resources, and changes in the climate of opinion. What is needed are mechanisms where Districts, FPCs and others can exchange views, and obtain information about what initiatives are being developed in other areas. The regions are well-placed to develop such mechanisms, which would not only assist FPCs and districts but also equip the regions to respond to local needs and make maximum use of small or large amounts of extra resources. At regional level information can be gathered, for example about different models of primary health care teams, types of collaboration between FPCs, DHAs and LAs, including the revised arrangements for involvement of FPCs in the planning and development of health services. Such a mechanism can create a climate for better co-ordination and dissemination of information which can in turn be fed by local knowledge.

Another group of questions centres on the extent to which initiatives deriving from the initial stimulus provided by the Acheson report and Acheson money can be sustained in the future. Use of extra money and various initiatives which were in response to Acheson have to be seen in the context of what else was happening and what their knock-on effect is. For example, buying cars for nurses is no more or less valuable than a research project into social deprivation or the use of an accident and emergency department; merely the parameters are different. On the other hand, establishment of a mobile clinic can only last if the long-term administrative and other support is provided and the initiatives are absorbed into long-term planning. Initiatives such as the purchase of road maps or computer software may appear minor, but the question is one of seeing how these assist in the overall planning of provision of primary care. The initiatives which are likely to be sustained are those which form a part of a whole and are not isolated or ad hoc. However, at this stage it is difficult to assess what impact, if any, the projects funded by Acheson money will have. What is clear is that these initiatives cannot be judged in isolation or individually. They are part of a process and would have to be seen in the context of each district's overall strategy. One-off initiatives are likely to be short-term and their impact short-lived.

Similarly, initiatives which were funded by other special funding, that is, King's Fund or Partnership money, but are within the spirit of the Acheson report, can only be judged on the basis of their long-term impact or what ripple effect they have had. For example, the appointment of a Primary Care Liaison Worker in Hackney, the establishment of Primary Care Development Projects in Tower Hamlets and Camberwell are all examples of short-term initiatives whose influence can only be sustained if arrangements and mechanisms which these projects have developed for better coordination are maintained. These projects are essentially filling the real need of bringing people together, particularly GPs who previously have been working in isolation, and drawing them into the planning process. If the lessons of these projects are to be sustained, then the arrangements should become part of the overall planning process. This to some extent is happening in Hackney where the joint working party on premises is now a permanent feature and beginning to take a strategic look at the question of premises. The job of the Primary Care Liaison worker is being phased out and its responsibilities taken over by the FPC and the Department of Community Medicine. Furthermore, what these specific initiatives have illustrated is that, apart from resources, the need at local level is to facilitate better exchange of information, develop effective working relationships and establish co-ordination between different people involved in primary care. Invariably it has taken a facilitator or a project worker to bring this about, who has taken action to alleviate or remove barriers which in the past have hindered collaboration. In other words, short-term projects which may appear marginal have to some extent helped the process of change.

Again, on the question of improvement of GP premises, the Acheson report provided the initial impetus, made the FPCs, the districts and local authorities more aware of the problems and encouraged them to work in collaboration with each other. However, some people have argued that because FPCs were reacting to criticisms they tended to support 'bad schemes'. It has been suggested that FPCs and others involved should have looked at the question of premises in relation to the whole pattern of provision in a given area and should have attempted to promote more group practices. This initial impetus may lead to more strategic planning in the long run, however, provided the arrangements which have been established for better co-ordination are sustained.

Moreover, with the recent reorganisation family practitioner services have been provided with an opportunity to plan strategically and adopt a more positive planning role. The presence of an active, enthusiastic, highly competent FPC, which perceives its role as an initiator and not a passive repondent, is equally essential. The establishment of FPCs as separate health authorities will require improvements to operational and planning links with other health authorities and suitable arrangements to ensure that FPCs can contribute fully to planning at regional and district levels. In this way changes inspired by Acheson can perhaps be further developed. The Report of the Joint Working Group on Collaboration between Family Practitioner Committees and District Health Authorities (April 1984) suggested development of FPCs' planning role 'to enable them to contribute a mutually acceptable Family Practitioner Service component to each District health plan'. It also proposed that FPCs should compile a Profile and Strategy Statement every five years and an annual programme.

Strategic planning involving both national and regional and local policies is indeed a key to future progress. While a great deal depends upon the attitudes of districts and FPCs, these can be facilitated in a much more coherent way if resource allocation, manpower planning, regional and national policies are in tune with local needs. The future long-term need is for planning activities to give greater priority and thought to the provision of primary care, not in isolation but in relation to local needs and general health services. The aim at the local level should be to get relevant information in order to assist planning; to create mechanisms for effective liaison and co-ordination between those involved in primary care and links between non-hospital and hospital services; and the training of GPs and nursing staff in practice organisation and simple management skills.

Equally, it is essential that the DHSS should actively encourage developments both in inner London and in other inner cities. In the first place, it could do more to promote the regional co-ordinating role in primary health care planning which has been suggested as one key to continued progress. There are already close and regular contacts between the Department and RHAs in relation to the hospital services. What is needed is greater recognition within the Department of the part which the regions can play in primary health care, and the development of corresponding mechanisms for strengthened contacts between the administrative and medical divisions concerned with primary health care and the regions.

Secondly, more might be done by the Department to overcome the obstacles to co-ordinated action on primary health care presented by the fact that FPCs are independent of RHAs and DHAs. The proposals by the joint Working Group on Collaboration between FPCs and DHAs are of course relevant here, but a more positive and sustained encouragement by the DHSS of collaboration in planning might be one way of improving the position. Given that there is now a much more direct relationship of accountability between FPCs and the DHSS, it is reasonable to expect the latter to assume a more positive line.

Finally, a particular problem in London remains: the split between four regions. The evidence of this study is that there is a need for some more permanent liaison mechanism rather than the various ad hoc devices which have been tried over the years. Clearly, the question goes further than the need for co-ordinating measures to improve primary health care in inner London, but if there were such a mechanism it could help to achieve a more effective response in London as a whole. Any initiative here would, as in the past, depend heavily on the DHSS.

These suggestions would, quite apart from their direct effect, also have the important consequence of providing an indication to health authorities and FPCs of the importance attached by the DHSS to improving primary health care in the inner cities. This in turn could help to stimulate local initiatives. The question of priorities is perhaps in the end the most important of all in looking to future possibilities. If local initiatives are to be sustained and developed, if the DHSS is to take a more active role, and if a worthwhile shift of resources into primary health care in the inner cities is to take place, then a higher priority than has so far been the case must be given to this aspect of the health services. The question of what prospect there is of this happening is bound up with likely pressures for action on this front.

There is, first, the possibility of pressures arising from the forthcoming Green Paper on primary health care. Whatever may be said directly about inner city problems in the Green Paper, it is possible the discussions generated by it may provide some impetus to the views of those who wish to give higher priority to the inner cities. On the other hand, if the paper is as wide-ranging as it has been rumoured to be, the inner cities will be only one of many issues clamouring for attention.

Secondly, there is the GMSC's study of under-privileged areas. If this leads the BMA to propose a different structure of payments to GPs, and this is accepted as the basis of future payments, there could be significant changes in the pattern of GP deployment in the inner cities. At the moment it is uncertain whether and when specific proposals will emerge, but one consequence will be that any such proposals will focus attention on primary health care needs in the inner cities.

Finally, there is the continuing evidence of problems in the inner cities, whether emerging from specific research such as that commissioned by the DHSS from the Department of General Practice at Manchester University, or from the experience of those who live and work there. This is likely to remain a constant factor, as it has for many years now, unless and until a sustained improvement in primary health care in the inner cities takes place.

Something has, therefore been done in response to Acheson. More remains to be done. More to the point, a good deal could be done now even within current resource constraints both centrally and locally, and, preferably, by both acting in consort. But primary health care in the inner cities must be given a higher priority if effective and lasting results are to be achieved. Without that, modest progress now and in the future is all that can be expected—small comfort for those whose life and work makes them only too well aware of the deficiencies in the primary health care services in the worst of our inner city areas.

References
[1] See Gerald Rhodes, *Committees of Inquiry*, RIPA/Allen and Unwin, 1975, pp.210-2.